PUFFIN BOOKS

HAPPY HABITS

DR ALEX GEORGE

HAPPY HABITS

7 STEPS TO BUILD A HAPPY LIFE

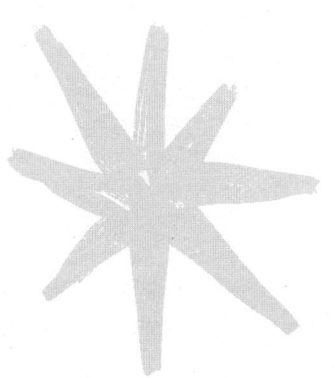

PUFFIN

PUFFIN BOOKS

UK | USA | Canada | Ireland | Australia
India | New Zealand | South Africa

Puffin Books is part of the Penguin Random House group of companies whose addresses can be found at global.penguinrandomhouse.com.

www.penguin.co.uk   www.puffin.co.uk   www.ladybird.co.uk

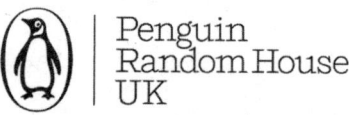

Penguin
Random House
UK

First published 2025
001

Text copyright © Dr Alex George, 2025
Illustration by Dynamo Limited
Additional material and research by Oscar Millar and Emma Young

All brands referred to in this book are trade marks belonging to third parties.

Text design by Dynamo Ltd

Printed in Great Britain by Clays Ltd, Elcograf S.p.A

The authorized representative in the EEA is Penguin Random House Ireland, Morrison Chambers, 32 Nassau Street, Dublin D02 YH68

A CIP catalogue record for this book is available from the British Library

ISBN: 978–0–241–77146–4

All correspondence to:
Puffin Books
Penguin Random House Children's
One Embassy Gardens,
8 Viaduct Gardens, London SW11 7BW

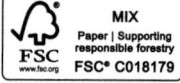

*I dedicate this book to every child
in their pursuit of happiness.*

HAPPY HABITS

WELCOME

I'm Dr. Alex, and this is my book *Happy Habits*, an introduction to all the **small things** you can do **every day** that make **big things happen**. Thanks for opening up this book, and well done — reading's a *great* habit to get into.

It's not an instruction manual and it's not a schoolbook, don't worry! What I want to share with you are what I call Happy Habits. They are a set of ideas I use that I think would help everyone spend their time in ways that will make all their dreams come true.

Neil Armstrong, the first person who walked on the Moon, was once a kid who made a habit of concentrating in his science class. Any rugby player you can think of would have made a habit of throwing and catching whenever they could. Taylor Swift will have sung in the shower.

And they did it again. And again. And again. Each time they got better, and things got easier. Their happy habit became their happy life. Their dream didn't just become a reality – **their reality made their dreams COME TRUE**.

So that's why I wanted to write this book. To show you how the happy little things you do today are what helps make a happy life.

So let's get started. Just getting started is one of the best habits we can have.

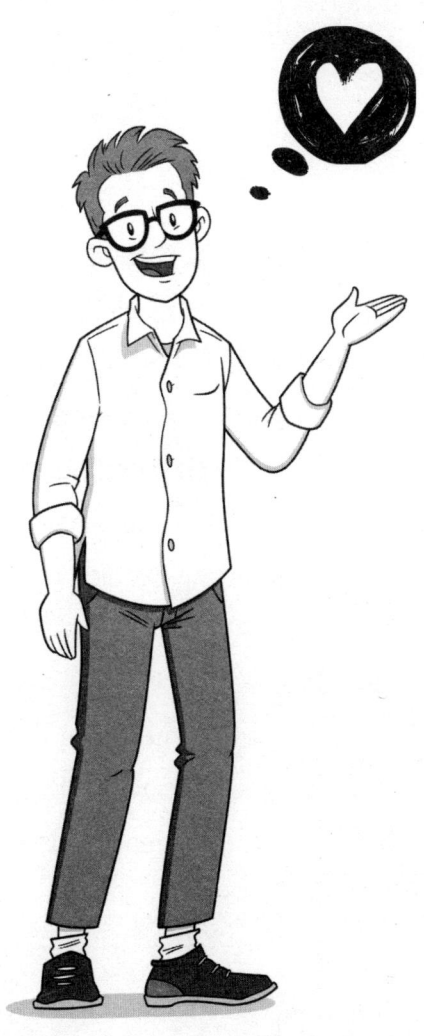

INTRODUCTION

WHAT DO YOU DO BEST?

If you had to think of something that you enjoy, that you are good at, and that makes you feel proud of yourself, what would you say?

I would say I feel good at running because I have trained for a marathon, or that I know lots of facts about the human body because I studied to become a doctor.

Maybe you are good at scoring goals. Or drawing horses. Maybe you're good at remembering the names of thousands of items in *Minecraft*. Think of that thing you have become good at.

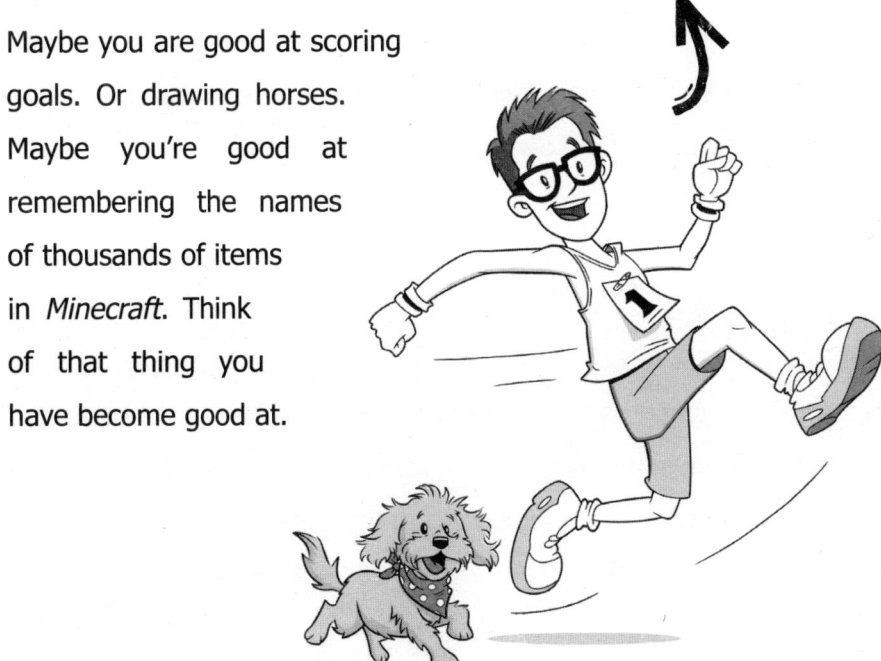

How do you feel when you are doing it?

Pretty good.

How do you feel about the fact that you *can* do it?

Proud.

And were you always able to do it?

No. I got better over time.

You see, we all have skills that we are proud of, that make us feel happy and that we got better at over time. The question is, how did we get better? And if we want to discover *other* things to enjoy and be proud of, how can we learn to do them?

The answer is – you guessed it (it's in the name of the book!):
HABITS.

A habit is something that we do often. It is also the **best way** to get better at something. So you found a habit – shooting footballs, drawing manes or remembering dragon eggs (I *think* that's from *Minecraft* . . .) and you did it a few times a week for a few years.

In that time, you went from being someone who could only kick a ball a few metres to someone who could take a corner.

You went from someone who could draw the outline of a horse to someone who could make it look pretty realistic.

You went from knowing about one item, to ten, to a thousand.

You formed a habit, and your habit made you happy because you learned to like doing it. Then, you felt proud of what you could do. I'll bet then that your habit probably didn't feel like something you had to remind yourself to do. You saw a football and would just start playing, or noticed your brown pencil and thought, *Time to draw a horse.*

It was *automatic.* This means that, unlike chores, you didn't need a big reminder or encouragement to do it. It just sort of happened, and as you got better, you felt more confident and more excited to do it again and again and again.

Because the best habits are automatic. We have to think about doing them for a bit but then, soon enough, we start doing them without even thinking. I want to tell you how you can make lots of good habits automatic.

Once we make our happy habits something we do without thinking, there is no question of how far we can go.

HOW FAR DO YOU WANT TO GO?

So you've thought about the things you have already improved at.

I'm guessing you have only had a couple of years to develop these skills. But you must have started to feel pretty good with the practice you've had – you should do!

Now imagine that rather than five years of practice, you've had twenty. Or instead of six months, it was sixty YEARS. That's a lot of goals or drawing or gaming! By the time you're done, you'll probably be scoring from the halfway line or creating life-size horse sculptures that look real.

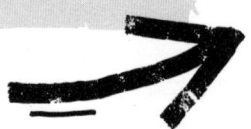

The habits you start or continue today could result in some amazing happiness and unbelievable levels of skill in your future. So if you can, don't imagine the future as some faraway time when you are old and grizzly – think of it as a moment that begins today. The future is the version of you that is getting better, starting from right now.

So let's think about what you would like to be able to do _someday_.

LET'S DRAW A PICTURE OF THE FUTURE YOU.

➡ Would you like to be happy? Someone who laughs a lot?

➡ What would you like to do for a job?

➡ What skills would you like to have?

Adults always ask kids the question, 'What would you like to be when you grow up?' so you might already have an answer. But what they _don't_ usually ask is what are you doing **today** to make that happen.

Successful inventors aren't at the top of their field because they said, 'I want to be a successful inventor' – they are there because they have developed their ideas, tested them and worked to make them the best they can be over time (sometimes years!).

The things you will achieve in your life don't just magically happen when you're a grown-up. They happen when you keep improving at some things from when you are a child because you have formed a habit.

You don't *become* a footballer on the day you score in the Premier League – you *become* one on the day you decide to start practising like one.

Say, for example, you answered the questions above like this:

➡ **Would you like to be happy? Someone who laughs a lot?**
Yes . . . and yes . . . LOL! (Sorry. I was just practising laughing – it's a good habit!)

➡ **What would you like to do for a job?**
I would like to be a marine biologist

➡ What skills would you like to have?

I would like to be able to scuba-dive.

OK, so you want to be a **healthy**, **happy**, **laughing, scuba-diving marine biologist**.

Great choice. But how do you become one?

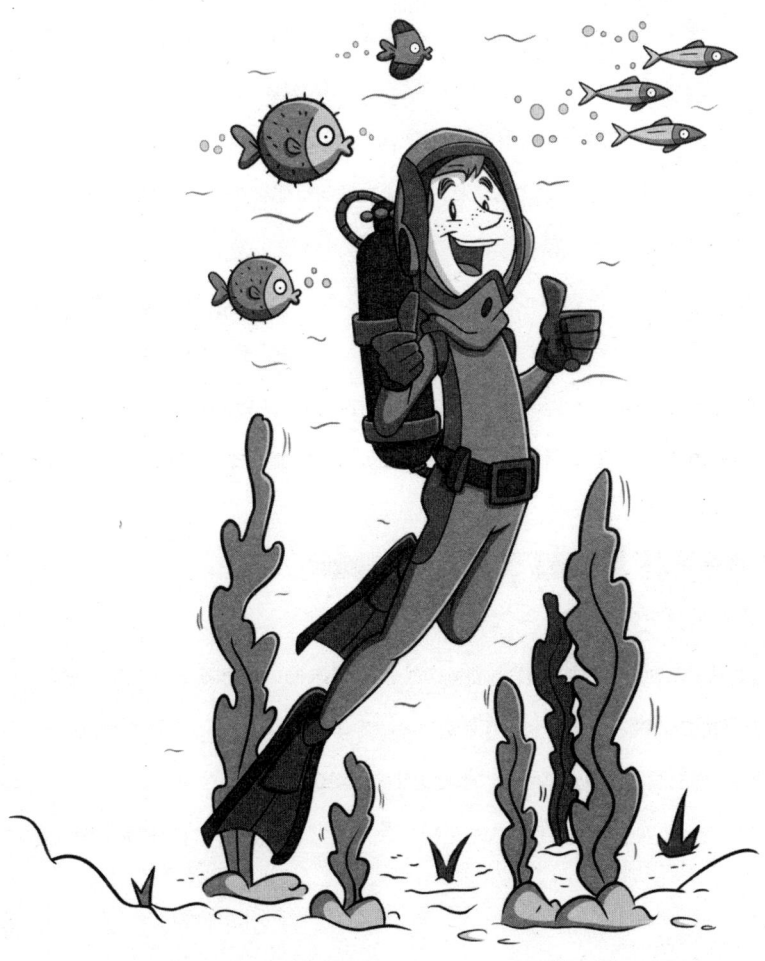

Well, this book is split into seven separate sections: **Move**, **Nourish**, **Rest**, **Plan**, **Joy**, **Connect** and **Breathe/Reflect**, with each section containing inspiration and advice on how to pick up small habits that grow into the bigger ones that make us happy – because **who you want to be *someday* is a result of what you do *today*.** Nothing massive, nothing hard – just finding little habits that make you happy and help you grow.

So, to become a marine biologist, you might need to take small daily habits from each section to help you work towards that goal. This might look like planning how you're going to learn all the fishy facts and nautical know-how you'll need, or making sure you're getting enough rest to keep your body and brain in tip-top shape – whatever feels good to you!

But before we get too far into how picking up these happy habits works, let's just read that last bit again:

Whatever feels good to you.

Every single person on this planet is unique. There may be sections of this book that you don't connect with, or which you need to adapt in order to suit your individual needs – this is especially true if you have either a physical disability or a neurodivergence diagnosis, such as ADHD, dyslexia, autism or dyspraxia. If some of the advice or habits listed in this book don't feel good to you, it's absolutely fine to park them for now and try something else. I'd always suggest talking through anything you are finding challenging with your grown-ups or healthcare team though, to see if there are strategies you can put in place to get the best from these happy habits.

We will talk in more detail about how happy habits work in each section, as I know that right now it might sound like a lot of things to put together. But the cool thing is that **every few minutes you spend on a habit you enjoy makes that habit even more effective and even easier the next time.**

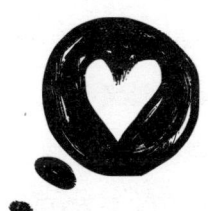

WHY I WANT TO TELL YOU ALL THIS

Because happy habits changed my life, and when I was a kid, I didn't really understand how helpful they could be.

I used to think you were either a person with good habits or a person with bad ones. You can probably guess which one I felt like most of the time.

School was really hard for me. I struggled to sit still and concentrate. Reading and writing were difficult, and I never finished my work on time. It made me feel left out and different from my classmates. I became shy and too scared to get involved in things I would really have liked to do, like playing sports or going to birthday parties.

I mostly felt worried. A LOT. I worried that my teachers thought I wasn't good enough. That my parents thought I was lazy. That the kids in my class didn't like me. I didn't know what to do, and I didn't think there was anything I could change. Whenever I was told off for a 'bad habit', like doing my homework late or having too much screen time, I just thought it was another sign that people didn't think I was good enough.

I thought that good habits just sounded boring. Eating vegetables, going to bed early and making sure my homework was done on time all seemed like the opposite of fun. They seemed like they were just things getting in the way of having a good time or being happy.

This meant I felt stuck. I felt bad. I didn't have any good habits, and no one had explained to me that habits might just be the thing to make me feel better.

I felt worried that people thought I was lazy, and I felt sad when I got lower marks than my classmates. But I also *didn't want* to do hard work, and I didn't believe I could get better marks. So, I thought I would always be disappointed and that it was just my personality. I thought I would never find habits that worked for me and that I would always be someone who let himself – and other people – down.

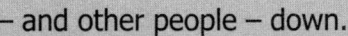

SPOILER: I WAS WRONG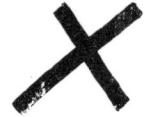

As it turned out, I was completely wrong. I learned that just a few small habits – nothing too hard – made the bigger ones feel manageable. Every little thing I did made the next one easier. Soon, the hard things in my life became easy. I started to do better, feel better and be happier.

> It became clear that I *was* good enough, and **habits** were a key part of that. **They weren't the *problem*; they were the *solution.***

I didn't need to worry about being lazy; I had to learn habits which helped me work better and smarter. I didn't need to worry about playing sports – I had to give them a try and learn how happy they could make me.

I realized that habits weren't *hard* things, but *happy* ones. Small changes that add up to big things. In my personal life and through my work as a doctor and mental-health ambassador, I've realized that developing the right habits in the right way is an amazing tool for our well-being. Repeatedly 'doing' a helpful habit is good for us now, but also helpful for next time because a habit gets easier each time we do it.

As our habits get easier to do, they become something we don't even have to think about. Do you have to think about getting dressed?

OK... SO I'M OUT OF MY PYJAMAS. ERRR... WHAT DO I DO NOW?!

No – you have done it so often that it comes naturally (though you might have to give a bit more thought to what you're actually going to wear!). As a result, you can do other things *while getting dressed* – you can sing, have a chat or think about the world's smallest cat (her name is Lillieput, and she is a breed called a 'munchkin'). When an activity or behaviour becomes a habit, we make space in our minds to add things on top of it.

We can practise new skills, get better at old ones and feel proud of ourselves for choosing to do it.

But we have to remember, our **habits aren't about being good or bad**. They aren't right or wrong, lazy or perfect. Our habits are just about being happy. We all have an idea of the sort of person we want to be, and who we are is the result of our habits.

> We feel proud when we do something that feels hard now in order to get better in the future.

We won't always get our habits just right because no one is perfect. The best solution is to try to do the right thing for ourselves, our bodies and our minds with small, positive decisions. We don't need to try to be perfect though; we just have to try and be kind to ourselves, and then, bit by bit, step by step, we'll start becoming the best we can possibly be.

It takes time, but boy, is it worth it.

So don't worry if you start slowly. Don't feel guilty if you sometimes forget to follow your routine or have a bad day. The great thing about habits is that they are for a lifetime, and you have your whole life to see which ones make you feel good. You just have to try.

The first step is to think about who you want to be. The second is to think about what habits make someone like that. The third is to work out a way to make those habits *easy* to commit to and do *every day*.

Then, all you have to do is *live*. It's a great habit.

Let's start by thinking about how we form habits.

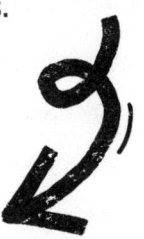

HOW HABITS ARE FORMED IN OUR BRAINS

Habits are formed when we do something enough times that it becomes automatic. Say, for instance, you want to start a new habit of drinking a small glass of water before bed. (I love to do this, as it helps me sleep better.) The first few evenings, you may forget and need reminding. But after you've had your drink a few evenings in a row, your brain will automatically start to remind you to fill up your water glass at bedtime, without you having to think about it. Amazing!

This applies to anything we want to build into our lives, so the possibilities are endless. The aim is to make our happy habits **automatic**, so we do them every single day but without much effort. Over the coming days, weeks and months, these happy habits could make a huge difference to your life.

Imagine learning a new language or sports skill. The hardest part is at the start when our brain finds the new task more challenging. This is temporary – we just need to push through and keep trying, because it always gets easier. Soon, with enough repetition it becomes easy and can even start being fun.

Habits are happy because, with some work, they make the hard things in life fun and fun things easier (as we don't have to spend so long thinking about how we will get things done).

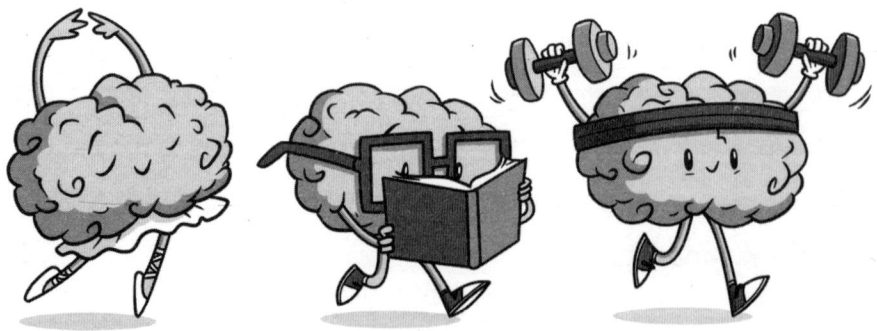

Even better, our whole brains are capable of something *amazing*, called **neuroplasticity**.

This is the brain's ability to change itself based on what we do and learn. The brain contains billions of tiny cells called **neurons**, which send each other messages. Each time a new message is sent, it creates a pathway in our brain. The more a certain pathway is used, the stronger it becomes. And this is why when we learn something new, it's hard at first, but the more we do it, the easier it becomes. Our brain is literally changing a tiny bit every time – and that's why our happy habits make lots of small changes that result in big, brainy progress.

As babies, this is how we learn to walk and talk, and it continues throughout our lives as we develop new skills.

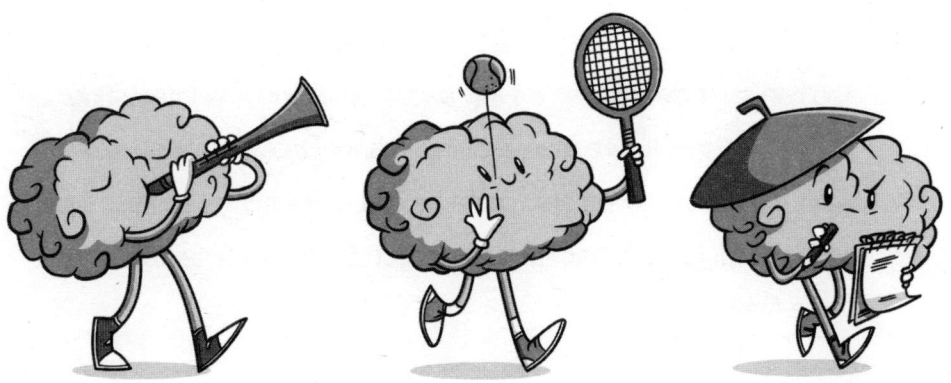

Your brain is always actively learning: the neurons are firing off messages, and the pathways are getting stronger the more you do something. The possibilities are endless, so imagine them.

CHOOSE YOUR OWN HAPPY HABITS - AS MANY AS YOU LIKE

In this book, we're going to be looking at all sorts of habits. Habits to do with movement, creativity, friendships, nature and more. The habits you want to focus on should be connected to how *you* want to live. The way *you* want to feel, the things *you* want to be able to do and the life *you* want to have. All of the habits in this book are just as important and valid as each other, and some may feel more relevant to you and how you want to live than the rest. All of which is absolutely OK! Just remember that progress doesn't always happen in a straight line though, so if you have a bad day, a bad week or even a bad month you can always start over again.

You can start by focusing on any section that you find interesting. If you are the future scuba-diving marine biologist, you might want to look at movement (gotta be a good swimmer to keep up with the dolphins) and planning (got to make time to study those fish!) first.

But choose whichever works for you – **building new habits is a personal thing**. Once you get the hang of one or two and you've got into the habit of creating new habits, you can try some others. You'll be able to apply everything you've learned about habits themselves to whatever new skill you want to develop.

Because it's the start of a journey that could take you *anywhere*. It starts with the step of deciding to make a habit of good habits, and it ends up wherever your dreams are.

So say it with me: I'm ready to make my dreams come true, a little bit at a time, with happy, healthy habits.

Let's go.

Oh . . . you can take off the flippers; you don't need them right now.

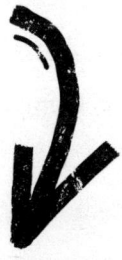

PART 1: MOVE

HAPPY HABIT 1: MOVEMENT AND EXERCISE

I really believe movement – in whatever form you can manage or enjoy – is crucial for our overall well-being and happiness.

It's important to say here that there is no 'right' way to move your body – it's all about what feels good and is manageable for you. Everyone's bodies are different and not all bodies work in the same way. If you have a physical disability for example, you might need some adjustments to help you with movement and exercise or help from experts such as physiotherapists. That could be special equipment like a sports wheelchair, adapting a team game to be more inclusive or working together to improve your range of motion. You can speak to your grown-ups about how best to make movement work for you.

Whether you love to run, move to music or play, you might not realize that because they make your heart beat faster, all of these count as exercise. Scientists all over the world have studied exercise and consistently found it is incredibly good for our bodies as it:

➡ builds healthy bones. Activities like running and jumping puts our bones under pressure and makes them stronger.

➡ strengthens our muscles. If you have noticed that you can run faster each year as you grow older, jump higher or go further, it's probably because your muscles have grown.

➡ improves our flexibility. Perhaps you know someone who does gymnastics, or who can do the splits. This is the result of a good habit of exercise. The more you make a habit of strrrrrrrrretching your body out in a gentle and controlled manner, the more it will be able to move safely and strongly into different positions.

➡ boosts our hearts and immune system. This means that every time we get our body moving, we protect ourselves from getting poorly – which is often the *only* reason not to exercise or play.

This all sounds pretty good, right? Well, even better, **it can even improve our *minds*!** Incredibly, exercise and movement can make us better at our studies by helping us be more focused and able to complete harder tasks. (While some gentle movement may help some brains to focus, try to hold off on doing a full dance routine as you're doing your maths tests, or the paper could go flying!)

Exercise improves our brain function because it allows more blood to flow to our brains. Have you ever ridden an old bicycle or seen a machine where the parts were rusty so it moved slowly? This is because there is friction in between those parts, which means they don't move quickly, and so sometimes people add oil to a machine to make it move smoothly. Exercise kind of does the same thing – it smooths out our mind, allowing blood to flow to our brain and our thoughts to connect and process better. You don't need to go to a mechanic to get your brain moving though – you just need to get your body moving.

Trying out a new sport can also help you become better at things in your day-to-day life – for example, wheelchair basketball can help wheelchair users improve their chair control and learn new tricks for navigating everyday spaces, while kicking a football around with your mates helps improve spacial awareness and teamwork skills. Win-win!

It can also make you happier, not just because you enjoy the activity, but because your body releases **endorphins** when you get moving. Endorphins are hormones that humans initially developed as a sort of natural painkiller, and as a result they make us feel relaxed and happy. If you've ever had that nice warm fuzzy feeling after going swimming or playing sport, that's the feeling of endorphins.

Another hormone that gets released is **dopamine**. This is often called the 'reward hormone' – a sort of prize that our body gives us for exercising. It exists because our body wants to say well done, and also to encourage us to do it again. This goes way back to when we had to hunt for our food, and a bit of encouragement to get up and run after a mammoth was *pretty handy.*

That's why we actually get *more* energy when we exercise. Unlike a car, which runs out of fuel as it moves, humans actually get re-energized by movement. So we're more energized, focused and fitter thanks to this healthy habit. Best of all, both endorphins and dopamine make us feel happy, and that's what makes exercise such a happy habit.

LETTER FROM A CAVEPERSON

Dear Future Person,

I am very jealous. I hear that you can get fruits, vegetables and meat from something called a chop . . . sorry, a shop. Then you put it in a magic box (a hoven?), and it becomes hot and ready to eat. That is incredible, and I can't wait to live in the future. (Hang on, I have to wait how long?!?)

I have to chase a mammoth for my dinner, probably for miles. Once I catch it, I have to drag the meat back. Then I collect nuts and berries from the area around my house cave.

I'm really not in the mood today. I wish I could just stay at home and do some cave painting. At least I know that after I chase that mammoth, I'll get a nice feeling in my body. I'll be tired, I'll be hungry, but I'll feel a warm glow that stays with me until I get home.

If I didn't have that feeling, I probably wouldn't even bother. I'd just get a take away — by which I mean I'll take something away from the cave next door. Which is never popular.

Anyway, I've got to run . . . after a mammoth and AWAY FROM THAT SABRE-TOOTH TIGER.

It's gonna feel good.

Best,

Caveman Carl

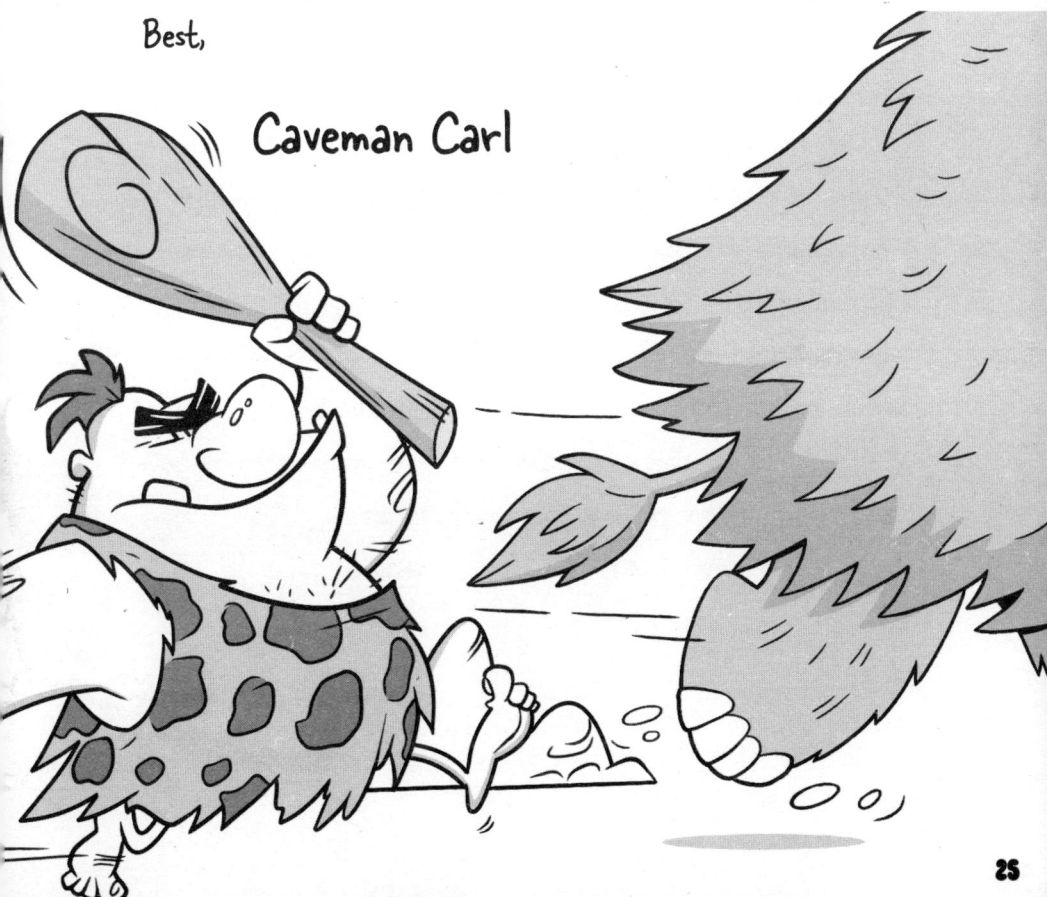

Dopamine (the reward chemical) is also great because it **makes us feel relaxed and less likely to worry**. The dopamine our body creates from exercise makes us feel restful. I know what you're thinking – aren't exercise and rest opposites? You're right, but that's why they work together. When we *finish* exercising, our body sends us a message to say, *well done, you've tired me out; time for a rest.* This is a feeling that makes us relax, but it also helps us focus less on the things that worry us.

We are less likely to worry after exercise, and *definitely* less likely while we exercise. This is because a worry is a focus on something that *might* happen, but exercise gives us something interesting and challenging that *is* happening, and we tend to prioritize what we are doing in the moment. Try worrying about a test while doing one hundred star jumps or racing after a ball! You'll find that your mind *prefers* concentrating on the exercise because, unlike the worry, focusing on what is happening at the moment is helpful and fun.

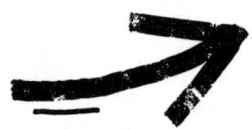

Then, at the end of all that, **you sleep better too**. If you've ever fallen asleep in the car after an energetic day (or after chasing a mammoth if you're Caveman Carl), you'll know what I mean.

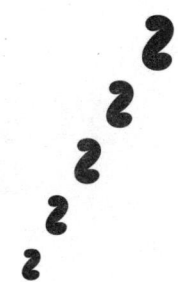

So, if you already enjoy exercise, see if you can make it into a habit – something you decide to do *every day.* If you don't enjoy it yet, see if you can try out some different ways of getting moving. You'll not only feel great but also more confident, because every time we decide to do something new, we realize we are capable of learning and growing.

It might be uncomfortable for a bit, but try to remember that doing hard things is only uncomfortable because we are trying hard and learning. It's not a sign that something is wrong, only that we are pushing ourselves to grow and get better.

Best of all, each time we get through the hard part of picking up a new habit, we grow more confident that we can do it again next time.

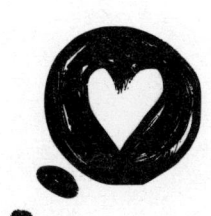

FIVE FUN FACTS ABOUT THE HUMAN BODY

1   The word 'muscle' comes from a Latin term meaning 'little mouse' – this is what the ancient Romans thought a bicep muscle being flexed looked like! Two tickets to the mouse show!

2   On average, your heart will beat more than three billion times during your lifetime. Beat that!

3   Keep having strange dreams? Our brains are sometimes more active when we're asleep than when we're awake.

4   Your lungs aren't the same size. Your <u>left</u> lung is a little smaller than your right one in order to make space for your heart (awww).

5   Your amazing spine (or backbone) is made up of 33 small bones called vertebrae. As you age, some of these fuse together, explaining why the average adult only has about 24.

Hi, it's me, **FUTURE YOU!** Thanks for moving around — you've made *me* healthier every time you've run, danced or worked up a sweat. I'm doing great, because the things you start doing now are things I get to be really good at later! I couldn't do it without you . . . errr, I mean . . . me.

P.S. Remember your PE kit next Friday and start learning to do cartwheels — the sooner you start, the better I'll be.

FUTURE YOU

GETTING STARTED

But what if exercise is *the last thing* you want to do? Maybe it feels too hard, too embarrassing, or you don't know where to start. Maybe you don't enjoy PE lessons at school much and feel a bit worried about taking up a new sport outside of school. I'd always suggest talking to the trusted adults in your life as the best way to help you get started.

When you've done that, take it a little at a time. As I've already said, everyone who is now a karate sensei was once a kid going to their first lesson, and every Paralympic cyclist once sat in the saddle for the first time.

Start by thinking of something you would like to do. If you've been inspired to try a cool-looking activity that you'd like to be good at *someday,* take the first small step today by considering how to get involved.

Ask an adult to help you find out where you can do it, and maybe see if any of your friends would be interested too. Then decide when you'll go to the place where it's happening, just to have a look or to give it a try.

Let's say the thing you'd like to try was **skateboarding**. This might mean going down to a skatepark and watching the older kids doing their tricks. This will give you an idea of what you could do in the future. Maybe they will let you have a go at standing on their board to see what it feels like. People who love to do certain things *also* love encouraging other people to give it a try.

Or perhaps you'd like to try a new style of movement – let's say **chair yoga**. You could look up a video on YouTube, and then try and safely copy a few of the easier poses. Even if you're just doing an impression, you'll get the feeling of what it would be like to practice yoga!

The key is that you give it a go, and don't worry about doing it perfectly or getting it wrong. We all *have* to get new things wrong to get better – it's part of how we learn. Focus on congratulating yourself for showing up and doing it, even if it's only a five-minute stretching session, a visit to the skatepark or signing up for a class.

IF YOU'VE MADE A START, GIVE YOURSELF A HIGH FIVE.

When you see how good making a start feels, you'll have even more encouragement to keep on going! Then you can do it as much or as little as you like.

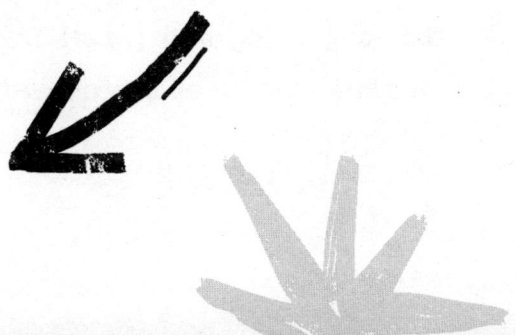

NHS guidance advises that young people between the ages of five and eighteen should do at least 60 minutes per day of physical activity. This should be a mixture of *moderate* activity that makes you feel a little bit out of breath and *vigorous* activity that really makes your heart beat fast. Sometimes it might just be walking or riding your bike, and other times it could be running or swimming.

This guidance varies a little for children and young people with a disability, however, who are advised to do 20 minutes of physical activity a day (splitting it into smaller chunks of time if needed). Challenging but manageable strength and balancing activities are also really important and should be practised three times a week.

It's better for our bodies to spread our exercise out throughout the day, so that we never spend too long being still (apart from when we're sleeping – no 'sleep skateboarding' please!).

If you'd like to try something new, but are feeling nervous, try it once. If you decide it's not for you after trying it, no problem! You'll have learned something new and confirmed just how brave you can be.

MAKE IT YOUR OWN

There are so many activities to choose from, including team sports like wheelchair football, classes like ballet or street dance, or exercise you can do on your own, like walking, swimming or home workouts. I like to keep fit with a variety of exercises, including stomping (brisk walking), running, football and tennis, so that I don't get bored of just doing the same one.

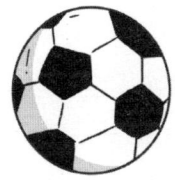

Keep looking until you find what you really enjoy! I gave jujitsu a go but realized I preferred other sports – particularly ones where I got to be outside rather than in a sweaty room.

Mix up your exercise in different seasons. I love to play tennis in the summer, but when it's cold, I prefer going to the gym inside. For a long time, I didn't go to the gym because

I felt worried I would look silly lifting weights. Then, after I tried it once, I realized that we never look silly if we are trying our best, and even if I did, people are there to get stronger, not to judge me. Adding that new habit didn't just make me fitter but more confident too.

Remember, **you can always change your habits**. Maybe it's taekwondo this year and swimming the next. It's extra helpful to try different types of movement because the more different things we try, the more our brain adapts and learns.

In the end, you get to choose what you enjoy and you should be proud of that. Some people prefer exercising on their own, focusing their mind and seeing if they can get better than they were yesterday. Others prefer being part of a team because you also get to make friendships as part of your exercise experience. This can be great because making friends and being part of a community is something that makes us even healthier and happier than just exercising on its own.

So maybe try both team sports and individual exercise to see which works for you. Maybe you'll like them both, which is great. As I said, any one kind of movement will help your body and brain improve one another.

> Let's start this habit today! Get a calendar and start ticking off all the days you exercised, then you can feel proud when you look back and see what you've achieved.

DR ALEX'S FAVOURITE HABIT

I am training for a marathon (26.2 miles)* at the time that I'm writing this book, which means loads of running practice! But if you asked me my favourite way to get moving, I would say walking in nature.

I grew up in Carmarthenshire in Wales, and I used to love stomping in the mud and picking blackberries in the country lanes, as well as climbing trees. (When I was three, a man passing our house had to ring the doorbell to tell my mum that baby-me was in a tree outside!)

As I got older, I discovered running was another great way to get my heart rate going outdoors.

I even decided to do a podcast called *The Stompcast*, where I chat to a guest while taking a walk. It's great because we

---

* That's a *really* long way! You legally have to be over 18 to take part in an organized marathon though, so you definitely don't need to worry about running this much at your age.

both get some exercise and people feel more relaxed and chatty outside. Exercise makes us calm and so does nature, so together they make us feel great.

Even better, it's free and easy to do. You don't necessarily need any fancy equipment – just head outdoors! So whether you live in the country or a city, grab your grown-ups and pop into a park or green space for half an hour – it can be just what you need to clear your head.

NO SUCH THING AS WASTED EXERCISE

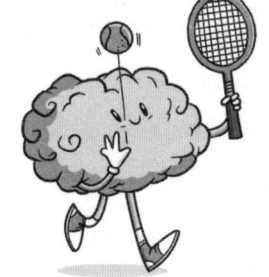

Remember, exercise isn't about winning. Although we sometimes play sports to win a medal or prize, that's really just a bonus. What matters is the joy of the experience and how it makes us feel.

Have you ever watched a dog running in the park? They aren't trying to win or worrying about how they look (the answer is usually very muddy). They just want to play and enjoy moving their body. Sometimes competitions are fun, but the real happy habit is learning to love movement in whatever way works for your body and feels good to you.

So just enjoy the moments and the movement. Races can be fun, and it can feel great to score goals or win prizes, but the real reason we exercise is because it makes us happy. If we know that then we have always won, no matter what the result.

TAKE A BREAK

Your body will tell you when to take a break and when to go faster. Some days you might need a rest, and during some exercises you'll need to take a break.

The more you practise this happy habit, the better you will understand how your body is feeling.

When I started running, I felt embarrassed to stop and walk sometimes. Then I realized I needed to do what was best for me, not worry about how I looked. Taking those breaks made running more enjoyable, and because it was enjoyable, I kept up the habit! Now, it's a part of my marathon training to walk sections of each run.

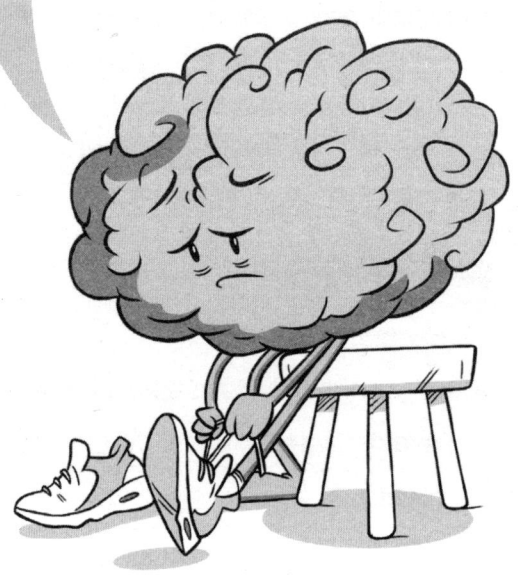

BUT I REALLLLLLY DON'T FEEL LIKE IT TODAY!

There are times when you can't, or shouldn't exercise. For example, if you're injured or unwell and your doctor has told you to rest. Some people may also have longer-term health conditions that mean they're not able to exercise for periods of time. Plus, sometimes we might just not have time – like when we're away on holiday and too busy eating ice cream by the pool. That's more than fine – it's good, in fact, as we all need to rest and recharge on a regular basis.

There will also be days when you just don't feel like moving! Everyone feels like this sometimes. The key is to remember how good you'll feel *afterwards*. You'll sleep better, and you'll feel happier and less anxious. Exercise helps boost our energy levels and puts a literal bounce in our step, so remember that a little bit of resistance is all that stands between you and great benefits.

So tell yourself that you'll do a small amount of movement, just to see how it feels. After five minutes, you can stop, but if you feel like you can carry on, try to do so. If you have a condition that means you need to be extra aware of your body, follow the guidance of your health team and your grown-ups.

Then by the time you finish, you'll be glad you did it. Your future self will be grateful to your past self for having a go, and you'll get even more confident in your ability to stick to your happy habits in a way that works best for you.

This is important because there will be a lot of times in your life when you have to do something you don't feel like doing. The more practice you have in getting going, the easier those times will feel, so **think of your exercise as life practice!**

A good workout can sometimes cause us to feel achy, which is usually a healthy sign that our muscles are getting stronger. It's not normal to feel *a lot* of pain during or after exercise, though, so stop what you're doing and check with a grown-up if you experience this. It may be that you are pushing yourself too hard or doing the exercise incorrectly.

If you have a disability, the same advice applies, but I also recommend using a service like 'Every Body Moves' to find great accessible sports and activities near you!

Athletes like cyclist Dame Sarah Storey, adventurers like sailor Ed Jackson and dancers like Rose Ayling-Ellis show that following a passion for movement really is for everyone.

HABIT HACK: HOW SMALL HAPPY HABITS CREATE BIG WINS

One reason that habits are great is that they give us something small to focus on. In the case of exercise, like sports or dance, we might have a big goal, like winning the World Cup or performing in front of thousands of people.

But while these are great things to dream about, they can seem a long way in the distance when we are starting out. Our habits let us focus on what we can do today.

The big goal is the *result* of the habit we have taken up, because each bit of practice or effort we put in takes us further.

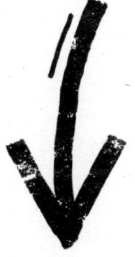

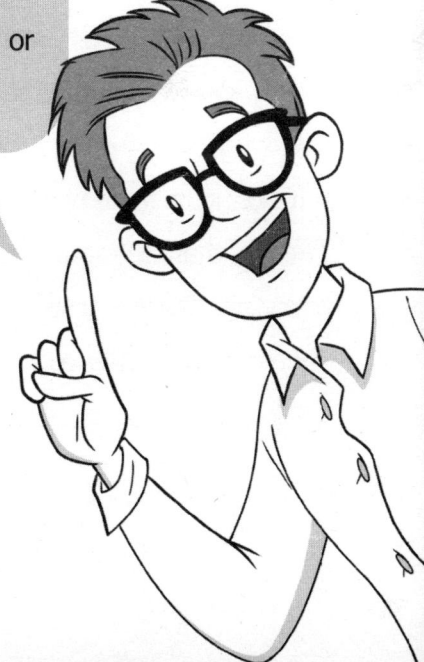

Imagine you were asked if you were capable of climbing a mountain. Starting out and looking at the very top, you might say,

That is too far, I can't do it.

But what if someone said,

Can you take one step?

You would say yes. When they asked if you could take another one, you would probably say yes again.

If you kept focusing on one step after another, you would realize that the mountain might have *seemed* too big to climb, but every step up it was possible. So, you were capable after all.

THE MAGIC OF REPEATED HABITS

Now wait, because it gets even better. Imagine that with each small step on the mountain, the length of your stride got longer, and you moved faster. The first step was hard and small, but the next was easier and you went further, on and on until each step was covering a **huge distance** (as if you had some sort of super-step that let you do one hundred steps for every one).

This is what happens with our habits. The leap you make from one level to the next grows even bigger every time.

Instead of your skills progressing in a line like this:

1 - 2 - 3 - 4 - 5 - 6 - 7

It is more like:

1 - 2 - 3 - 5 - 8 - 13 - 21

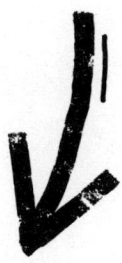

In the first sequence, we just move up one level at a time. But when we have a habit, everything we have already learned helps us progress faster on the next step. That means it's more like the second sequence because we start to learn and progress faster and better each time.

I want you to picture your skills like a tiny snowball at the top of a hill.

If you roll it just a little, it stays small. But if you keep rolling it, even just a little bit at a time, it picks up more snow and gets bigger and bigger. As it gets bigger, it can pick up even more snow than when it was smaller.

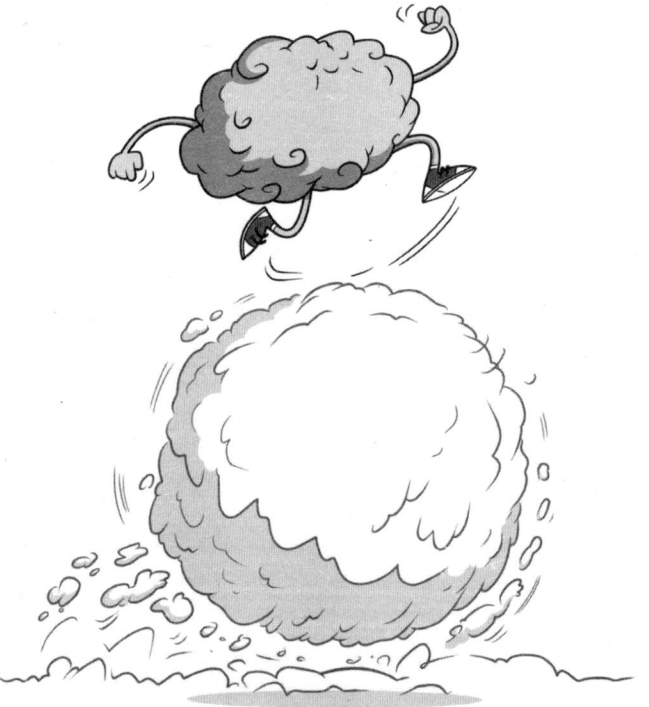

By the time it reaches the bottom, it's a giant snowball!

The bigger the snowball, the more snow it can add. The more days you have stuck to your habit, the more progress it will give you the next day.

Or maybe think of yourself when you first started reading and writing – you focused on learning how to hold a pencil, what the shapes of letters were and the names of numbers.

You didn't keep just getting better at reading the shapes of letters though. Soon, you were able to read whole words. Being able to read whole words means you can read a book. Reading books lets you find out pretty much any information in the world.

That small step of learning your letters ended up unlocking all the information in the world.

Because small habits lead to big changes.

PART 2: NOURISH

HAPPY HABIT 2: HEALTHY FOOD, HEALTHY BODY, HEALTHY HUMAN

'You are what you eat' makes it sound like you will turn into a digestive biscuit if you have one too many (could be fun . . . but probably not). In fact, what this phrase means is that how you feel and what you can do depends on the nutrition you give your body.

Some foods nourish and energize us – they make us feel healthy and buzzy, both mentally and physically – while others can make us feel tired and sluggish. I would never tell you to avoid a particular food, or that any food is good or bad. What is important is that we understand how foods make us feel and choose them based on whether they make us feel good now *and* stay healthy in the long-term.

It's all about building nutritious foods into our diets rather than restricting anything.

You can still enjoy your favourite treats here and there. For me, a cinema trip definitely isn't complete without some popcorn – half sweet, half salty.

We should think about what we eat and enjoy it without worrying. And one of the good things about not being a digestive biscuit is that we get to enjoy meals and snacks that help us grow!

So let's look at four of the main food groups that ideally we'd be building into each meal and try to understand a little more about them.

CARBOHYDRATES

Carbohydrates (or carbs) are food molecules. They give our bodies boosts of energy and help our brains function properly throughout the day. After we eat them, our bodies break them down into **glucose** (sugar) that is absorbed into our bloodstream and releases energy.

Carbs are found in starchy and sugary foods, including breakfast cereal, bread, pasta, rice, potatoes and sweet treats.

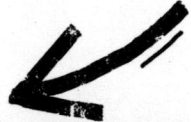

CARB FACTS

- Carbs are the body's main source of energy, giving you the get-up-and-go to run and play.

- They keep your brain sharp, like a high-powered computer.

- Athletes will eat starchy carbs like pasta to fuel a long training session, but often prefer a sweet carb like a piece of fruit for a quick boost before a shorter session.

FATS

Fats sometimes have a bad reputation, but they are a really important part of a healthy diet. They provide fatty acids – these are amazing for our skin health and immune system, which keeps us healthy by fighting off illness. They also provide energy and help us keep warm. However, not all fats are good for us, so if you can, it's worth spending some time learning more about them. However, as a very general guide, the healthiest types are those found in some meats, salmon, cheese, oil, avocados, nuts and seeds.

FAT FACTS

- About 60 per cent of the human brain is made of fats – and eating fats keeps your brain happy.

- Fats help us absorb vitamins A, D, E and K, which help our vision, immunity and circulation.

- Fats keep our blood pressure under control.

PROTEIN

Protein is another essential part of our diet. It is made of building blocks called **amino acids**. Different amino acids can combine in all sorts of ways to make all sorts of protein – and each protein has a different function in the body.

Some proteins repair muscle damage and help muscles grow back stronger. Some carry substances around your body. Others give structure to your cells. And antibodies are infection-fighting proteins!

We can find this amazing nutrient in lots of foods: meat, fish, eggs, milk, cheese, yoghurt, tofu, chickpeas, beans, lentils, nuts and seeds.

PROTEIN FACTS

- Most proteins contain at least 100 amino acids.

- If we didn't eat any protein, our entire body would swell up.

- Our hair is made of protein. Specifically, a protein called keratin, which also makes up animal fur and feathers.

FRUIT AND VEGETABLES

Getting your **five-a-day** is a popular phrase to remind us to eat at least five portions of fruit and vegetables every day. From blueberries and bananas to spinach and satsumas, fruit and vegetables are high in fibre, vitamins and minerals, which are good for heart health and keeping illness at bay.

Another reason to include plenty of fruit and veg in our diet is that they are great for supporting our **gut health** (the good bacteria in our digestive tract that boost our immune system and actively make us feel happy).

Scientists have recently found out loads of interesting stuff about gut health. It's wild to think that in your stomach you have **Tens of Trillions** of bacteria – and many of them are our friends! We need to protect these little guys because they affect the healthy function of our whole body – from our mood to our muscles. They love nutritious food like fruit, vegetables, fibre, wholegrains and live yoghurt. Ultra-processed food that isn't nutritious can damage them if we eat too much. It's important to remember that healthy eating is just about adding good stuff in, not taking other things out altogether.

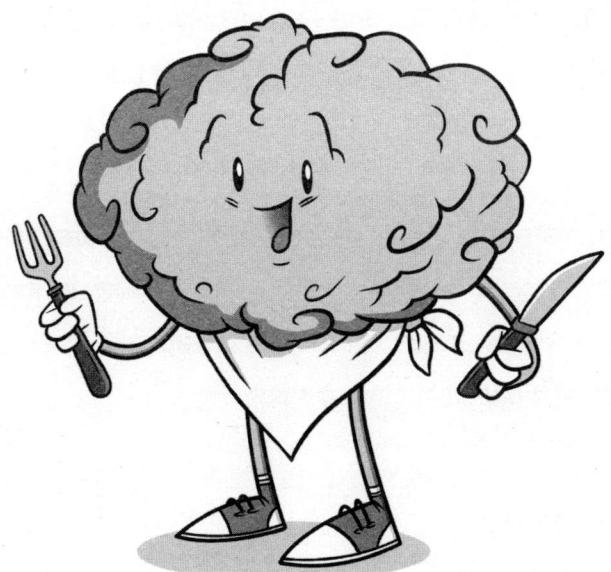

FEELING OVERWHELMED?

There's a lot of information out there about food choices, but we don't need to become experts or follow too many rules to make sure we eat well. Here are some easy shortcuts to healthy eating habits:

Eat the rainbow. A colourful plate will usually include all the key food groups and contain lots of vitamins and minerals. A beige plate isn't necessarily unhealthy, but colourful foods are more likely to be diverse and healthy.

Build in some **whole foods**. This means food that is in its natural state, grown on a farm, and hasn't been processed in a factory. This includes fruit and vegetables, nuts and seeds, beans and lentils, milk, yoghurt, wholegrains and unprocessed meats and fish.

Avoid too many **ultra-processed foods** – these are the opposite of whole foods and are prepared in a factory. They include snacks like crisps, ready meals, processed meats like ham, and any products with added sugars or salt.

It's *incredibly* difficult to avoid processed foods altogether. But balancing them out with whole foods is a great habit to get into. So if frozen pizza (a processed food) is on the menu for dinner, you can **balance it out** by having some whole foods like lettuce, tomatoes, sweetcorn, cucumber and a glass of milk on the side – with an apple for dessert.

Listen to your body. Mealtimes can be quite chatty, whether we're at school having lunch with our friends or at home with our family in the evening. So you'd be forgiven for not always paying full attention to what your body is signalling! Sometimes it will be craving something starchy; other times it might be asking for fruit. And it will definitely let you know if you are hungry, or if you've had enough food for now. Trust your body to tell you what it needs – over the noise of your sibling's terrible jokes!

CHALLENGE YOUR TASTE BUDS

It's important to enjoy your meals, and we all have our favourite foods that feel safe, comforting and delicious to us. Did you know that your **taste buds** (cells on your tongue that allow you to experience different tastes, like sweet, salty, sour and bitter) can change over time? This means that the flavours you enjoy might also change as you get older.

It's a good reason to keep trying new things, or things that you didn't like when you were younger. I used to absolutely hate olives and pickles, but now I love them, so I'm really glad I gave them another chance.

Get into the habit of trying one new flavour a week while continuing to enjoy your favourites. And if you don't like something now, give it another try in a couple of months.

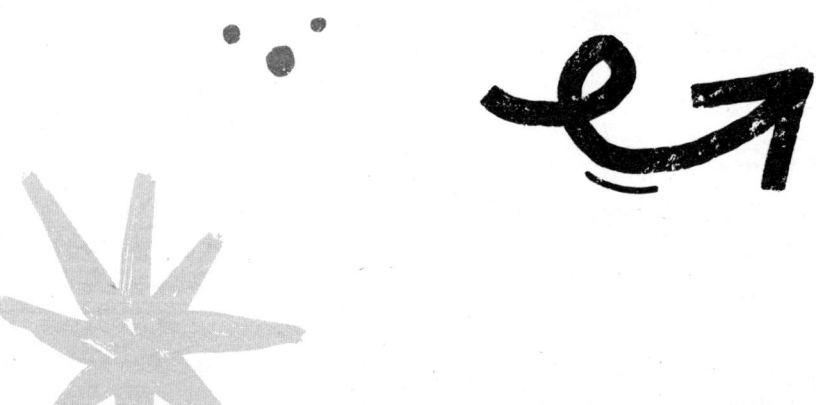

FUN FACTS ABOUT TASTE BUDS

- You can have between 2,000 and 10,000 taste buds – the number varies from person to person. 'Supertasters' are people with loads of taste buds, making them extra sensitive to bitter tastes.

- Your taste buds are replaced every two weeks!

- Taste buds can be found on the roof of your mouth, in your throat and in your oesophagus (the tube that transports food from your mouth to your tummy) – as well as on your tongue.

If someone offers you some food that you're unsure about, have a little nibble – you never know, it might become your **new favourite!**

FUTURE YOU

READY, STEADY, COOK!

Cooking is great, and preparing your own food is a really rewarding habit to get into. It can be fun and relaxing – and it's a great way of knowing exactly what you're putting into your body.

Cooking involves all of our senses – the **sights**, **smells** and **sounds** of the ingredients coming together, sizzling in the pan or roasting in the oven – and prepares our digestive system for the meal. This is why, while takeaways can be a handy treat once in a while, home-cooked food is often the most comforting.

To get into the habit of cooking, it's great to have the help of a trusted adult who can teach you some basics and discuss recipe ideas. Is there someone at home who enjoys cooking who you could team up with?

My mum and I used to cook a meal together every Sunday for the rest of our family. It was a lovely bonding activity, and she would teach me a new recipe each week. Some of my favourites were cawl (a delicious Welsh broth), lasagne, apple crumble and chicken-and-leek pie. Peeling potatoes and chatting to my mum is a great memory, and I still remember the warm glow of having helped prepare a comforting, nutritious meal for my family.

What kinds of food are you passionate about? Could you, once a week, **prepare a meal or snack for yourself and your family?** You could make smoothies or pancakes for breakfast or invent a new kind of sandwich. Or how about making jacket potatoes and coming up with three different toppings – delicious!

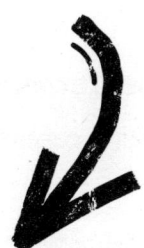

HAPPY HABIT 3: STAY HYDRATED

This one's an easy habit that doesn't require much effort but is excellent for your health. Water makes up more than **60 per cent of our body**, and keeping ourselves topped up is important for a variety of reasons:

➡ Your energy levels depend on your hydration.

➡ Your concentration depends on your hydration.

➡ Every single cell and organ in your body needs water to function.

➡ You don't want to turn into a crisp.
(OK, ignore that one.)

If that doesn't convince you that taking care of your water intake means taking care of yourself, here's a question.

WHAT HAS MORE WATER IN IT – A BABY OR A BANANA?

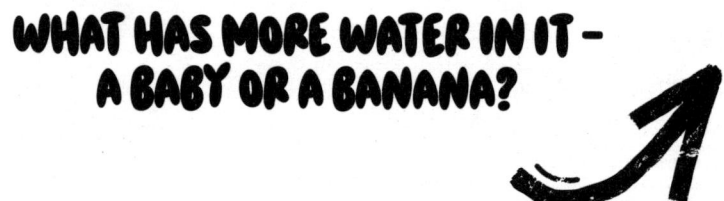

(Stop laughing. It's a serious question.)

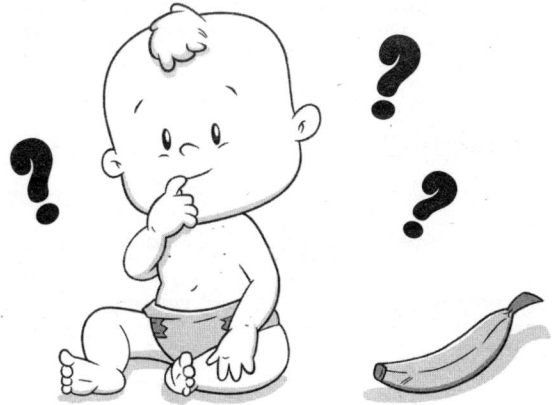

Correct: it's the baby. A baby can be up to 78 per cent water (wibble-wobble water-balloon baby!), whereas a banana is more like 74 per cent. An avocado is about 72 per cent, while a pea is similar to a baby at 78 per cent.

It is incredible how much water there is in a human body, but just as incredible is how much water other **solid objects** like fruits contain. A watermelon is 91 per cent water – it's almost magical that it doesn't end up sloshing all over the place!

If you want to learn more about this and really *see* the difference, ask your family if they will help you make some **dried fruit.** It's pretty easy and a great way to show how much water some fruits contain (as well as creating a great snack).

SIMPLE OVEN-DRIED FRUIT RECIPE

You will need:

> a selection of fruit – apples, pears, bananas, mango, kiwi, pineapple, strawberries, plums and peaches all work well
> a peeler
> a sharp knife
> some kitchen roll or a tea towel
> baking trays
> some baking paper

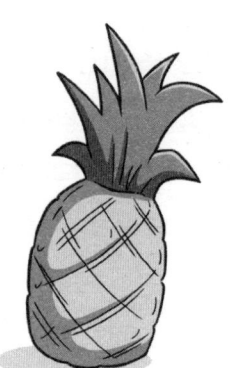

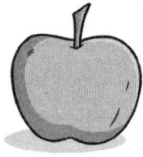

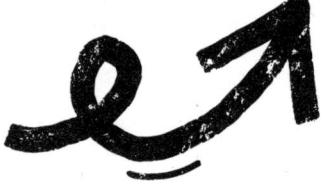

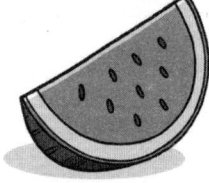

Method:

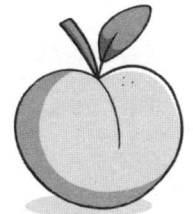

1. Preheat oven to 60–70°C.

2. Wash your fruit thoroughly.

3. Peel the fruit (if needed).

4. Ask an adult to help you slice the fruit evenly to create slices 3–5 mm thick.

5. Pat each slice dry using kitchen roll or a tea towel.

6. Line the baking trays with baking paper.

7. Arrange slices in a single layer so they are not touching, and place the trays in the oven.

8. Keep the oven door slightly open for airflow.

9. Bake for approximately 4–10 hours, depending on fruit (you will need to flip the slices halfway through).

10. When the time is up, check that the slices are dry but still slightly bendy.

What you will find is that the fruit pieces become *way* smaller and shrivel up, but they remain *really* delicious. That's because the water is gone but the sugars remain.

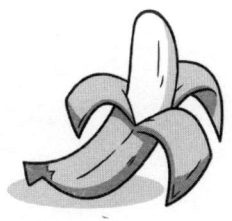

GIVE IT A TRY AND SEE!

So remember: stay hydrated, particularly when you do exercise that makes you sweat. Water regulates our body temperature by making us sweat when we're too warm, but it also keeps our brains and bodies alert and functioning correctly. It lubricates our joints, delivers oxygen around our body and makes our skin glow. **Hydration will make you perform better in every way.**

How can we know if we're drinking the right amount? Well, if you're drinking enough water, your wee will be pale yellow or straw-coloured. Any darker and you should probably drink some more. So learn from your pee . . . I mean it.

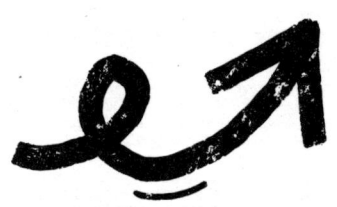

FUN WATER FACTS

- Nearly 71 per cent of the Earth's surface is covered by water.

- Up to 60 per cent of the human body is water, but don't worry, you can't burst – it's inside your cells.

- We are drinking the same water as the dinosaurs did – kind of! Water is constantly recycled by the Earth's water cycle (where it travels from clouds, down to the earth and then rises back up to become clouds again), so the water we drink today has been here for over 4.5 billion years in one form or another.

- Humans can only last for around three days without water (we can last much longer without food).

Just like anything, drinking water is a habit that will become easier to do the more you do it. Here are a few tips:

♥ Drink a glass of **water when you wake up in the morning**. It's normal to wake up feeling thirsty, because we often get slightly dehydrated during our sleep. A glass of water is the best way to wake your mind and body up before breakfast. Keep a special glass or mug by your bed to remind you.

♥ Drink a small glass of **water before bed**. You could do this before brushing your teeth so that it becomes part of your normal routine.

♥ Aim to drink **1.5 litres of water per day** (that's six to eight glasses). This might be more or less depending on your age, size and activity levels.

♥ Try filling a jug of water with some pieces of fruit (like lemon or cucumber) or herbs (like mint) and popping it in the fridge. This creates an extra healthy and **delicious flavoured water**. Which will help you to . . .

♥ **Avoid too many fizzy drinks** – they don't hydrate us properly.

♥ Drink more water in **warm weather and after exercise**.

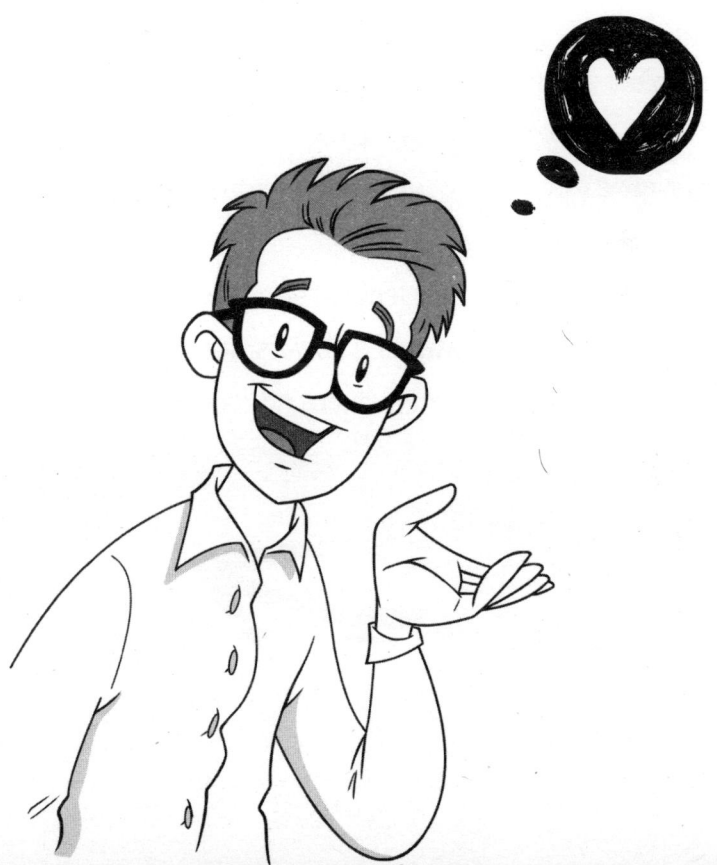

HABIT HACK: MAKING HEALTHY FOOD TEMPTING

We all *feel* like we are in control of our brains – we have thoughts, we make decisions and we get our body to act. We have to go to school, so then we think, *Where is my PE kit?* and we tell our body to move around and find it. Sometimes this takes longer than expected (*Who put my shorts behind the sofa?*), but it follows a pattern we understand.

But what if I told you that you are not *completely* in charge of your mind?

No, there's not some evil scientist controlling you from a lab or super-villains with mind-warping powers. It's just that our brains often respond to signals that we are not *consciously aware* of.

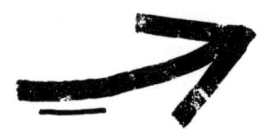

Say, for example, the way we all crave unhealthy food sometimes? For me, it's salty snacks – crisps mostly (though you might prefer sweets). Have you ever noticed that there are *certain times* or *certain places* that make you want sweets more than usual?

Maybe you have a regular movie night with your family, and you always get a chocolate bar. Now, *whenever* you watch a movie, all you can think about is chocolate.

This is called a **habit loop** (*Did someone say Hula Hoop?* No, we're not talking about crisps). It's like a little circle of behaviour that we can go through without even thinking about it.

We sit down to watch a movie, so we think of chocolate (because we are in the habit – this is called a **trigger**).

Then we want chocolate (this is called a **craving**).

We ask if we can have some chocolate (this is called a **response**).

We get chocolate, and we feel *chuffed* (this is called the **reward**), and next time it's movie night we think even more about . . . chocolate!

Somehow watching a movie led to chocolate without chocolate ever really being involved. We didn't see any chocolate or *decide* to want it, but watching a movie automatically led to it because we have formed a habit loop.

In this case, our *automatic* habit resulted in something that is not that healthy – chocolate – entering our mind. The cool thing is that we can use automatic habits to create healthy, happy habit loops instead.

So how could we create a habit loop for eating fruit? Well, you could start by picking something that you do all the time and creating an **attachment** to it – in this case, eating fruit. A good example of this would be to say, 'On my way home from school, I'm always going to eat an apple.'

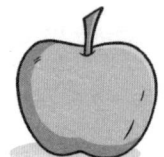

This is great because you're not going to *forget to come home from school* (that would be awful), and after you've had an apple on your journey a few times your brain will start **craving** one.

No evil villain manipulating your brain here! Just you, a happy, healthy scientist learning tricks that make you tick. Or maybe you create reminders that can act as **triggers.** You could draw a picture and put it up in your room (make it of a character you *don't* like). It could say, '**I bet you can't eat five pieces of fruit today**'.

Then, every day when you have had your five pieces, you can go up to the picture and say, '**Haha – I did!**'.

Now you have attachments and triggers, but you should also try to make fruit **tempting.** So pick some fruits you *really* like – think of your three favourites – and ask your family if you can always have them in the house.

Now you have a combination of:
- an attachment that means you always have fruit on your way home;
- a trigger that reminds you to have it at other times;
- tasty tempting fruits.

These three things should make the habit become easy. Now you just need to make it **satisfying.** So every time you say '**HAHA**' to your reminder picture, you could pop a sticker on it too. That will let you count the number of days that you have beaten the villain.

With these habit hacks you will have made your healthy fruit habit:

Obvious — with the picture on the wall and the routine.

Tempting — by picking your favourite fruits.

Easy — because it's in your routine.

Satisfying — because you get to say 'HAHA' to a picture and count the number of days you have won.

So our cravings can *actually become* good things because we can trick our mind into craving happy, healthy ones. Which I think is pretty cool.

We will talk about other habit hacks as we go on, but don't be surprised if you end up hiding bananas in places where you'll find them as another way to ~~trick~~ remind your brain to be healthy.

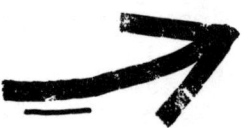

HAPPY HABIT 4: FRESHEN UP AND FEEL GOOD

How do you start your day?

Early mornings can sometimes be stressful – especially during the week when you're rushing to get to school on time. *Where on earth is my other shoe? Who left that banana in my bag?* (It was you – great habit hack!) *Why am I standing here staring at a picture of a villain telling me I won't eat five pieces of fruit?*

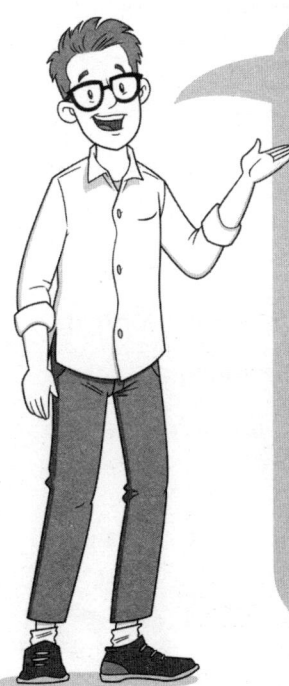

Starting your morning off right with a few simple tasks can set you up for the day ahead, no matter what you've got planned. While you probably already do plenty of the things we're going to be discussing in this chapter, the key is to learn how to move through them calmly and efficiently. As a result, you'll be less likely to forget things – and you can start each day feeling pleasantly prepared for whatever's ahead of you.

Just a reminder, though – as with all of the habits in this book, make them work for you. Read through the tasks listed on the following pages and then choose which order to do them in – there's no right or wrong here. You may prefer to tidy your room before showering, and that's totally fine! Also, feel free to add in your own morning habits – for example, feeding your pet (if that's something you're responsible for).

Once you've decided on the order, why not have a trial run at the weekend to see how long it takes you to do everything?

Then make sure you are setting your alarm at a time that allows you enough time to fit in your lovely new habits. Goodbye, last-minute drama. Hello, stress-free mornings.

BATHROOM BASICS

It's amazing how good it feels to freshen up. It's well worth the effort even if we're feeling tired, as it boosts our mood as well as keeping us clean and healthy. So here are a few things you can do every day to take care of yourself.

CLEAN YOUR TEETH

Unlike your baby teeth, which fall out, your adult teeth stay with you for life – so it's extra important to take care of them (just as you have with your baby teeth).

As we eat throughout the day, something called plaque builds up on our teeth. This is a sticky coating of bacteria that needs to be removed regularly by brushing. If the plaque isn't brushed away, we run the risk of tooth decay or gum disease developing over time. Brushing also keeps our breath minty-fresh.

Brush your teeth twice a day – ideally as soon as you wake up and then before bed.

Brush for at least two minutes each time – you can ask an adult to help you set a timer.

TOP TIP

My dentist friend says to gently polish your teeth with your toothbrush rather than scrubbing them. Pretend they are an expensive sports car that you don't want to damage!

FUTURE YOU ♡

Thanks for taking the time to brush our teeth. It can be so boring, and sometimes it's the last thing we want to do before bed. But fast forward ten or twenty years, and I've got some excellent news: our teeth and gums are in **great health**, we never get toothache, and the dentist is always happy with us at our check-ups. Phew!

SHOWER OR BATH

If we can, it's good to wash our bodies once a day, adding in a hair wash every two or three days as well.

Some people **shower** in the morning, while others prefer a **bath** or shower before bed, so choose whichever works best for you.

For an extra dose of freshness, you could try my 30-second cold water challenge by turning the shower to cold and letting the chilly water invigorate you. The cold temperature shouts **'WAKE UPPPPP!'** at your skin and your brain – helping you focus better for the rest of the day.

This is because cold water is an extreme stimulator of dopamine (our happy hormone). If you have a cold shower in the morning, dopamine levels rise in your brain and stay elevated for a number of hours, meaning you can have a really positive start to your day.

Even **ten seconds** will help – give it a try!

SKINCARE

Your face deserves some extra TLC – especially during puberty, which is the time when hormonal changes make our body grow up to be more like an adult's. These hormones can cause a whole range of issues with our skin, from eczema to acne to dryness. Here is a basic daily skincare routine that will help keep your skin feeling its best:

♥ Wash your face twice a day to get rid of dirt and oils that build up on the skin.

♥ Wet your face with lukewarm water and apply a gentle cleanser with your fingers or a facecloth. You can give yourself a relaxing massage at the same time by creating small circles on your skin with the tips of your fingers. Then rinse off the cleanser and pat your face dry with a towel.

♥ Next, apply a small amount of moisturizer to keep your skin nice and hydrated.

♥ Finally – and most importantly – in the morning, take time to apply some sunscreen with a **high SPF** (factor 50 or above). This is the best thing you can do for your skin, as the SPF reflects the Sun's damaging UV rays. Without the protection of SPF, there's a small chance that sun damage can lead to skin cancer in the long run.

Our skin's main job is to **protect our body** – from all kinds of things, including bacteria and extreme temperatures, so it's vital that we look after it.

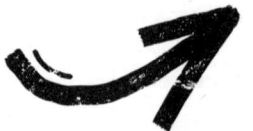

I'm so glad you're **slapping on the SPF** now. Loads of adults say they wish they had worn SPF from a young age, and they are right, because as kids our skin is even more vulnerable to sun damage. It's even more important because once our skin has sun damage, it's difficult to reverse the effects – so I'm grateful to you for staying **one step ahead** of those evil rays! The benefits to our health in the future are huge.

TOP TIP

Be sure to make SPF part of this skincare routine all year round, not just in the summer months. Do reapply more regularly when the Sun is out though.

If your skin is often sore or spots are making you uncomfortable, ask a grown-up to book you an appointment with your GP. They can be really helpful.

TOP TIP

BRUSH AND STYLE YOUR HAIR

Brushing your hair is actually good for the hair itself. It **stimulates the scalp**, which leads to healthier, stronger hair growth. So don't forget to spend a few moments in front of the mirror (or more than a few – it's totally up to you!).

PART 3: REST

HAPPY HABIT 5: BEDTIME HABITS TO GET THE BEST ZZZ'S

Another great day has passed. You've learned some new things, got your heart rate up and eaten all of your fruit and veg. Now you're ready for a good night's sleep. Simple.

Well, not necessarily. There's actually a lot to think about if we want to get into the habit of getting a good night's sleep. There are even sleep scientists who specialize in understanding the best ways to hit the hay! (They genuinely do research on things like pillow temperature.)

The main message from their research is that great sleep is **all** about habits. Our body has its own internal clock that tells us when to wake up and when to snooze, so if we can set that clock with consistent habits, half of our job is done.

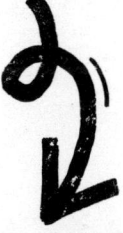

The other half is making sure that we create a pleasant, relaxing environment that *encourages* us to sleep. So turn off that heavy metal music, put down the remote and prepare to sink into a peaceful, relaxing . . .

Wake up! We're only *talking* about sleep – I need you awake for this bit. So, let's start by thinking about *why* we sleep.

IS SLEEP REALLY THAT IMPORTANT?

In a word: **yes**. A good night's sleep impacts our whole day, and a consistent sleep habit is key to our health throughout our whole life.

The quality of our sleep is about much more than just how we feel in the morning. **We learn better, move more efficiently and feel happier if we can get our rest right.** But don't worry, it's so easy, you could do it in your . . . *zzz*

Our sleep moves from light sleep (where you could be woken up quite easily) through to deep sleep and REM. The last two are where the magic happens.

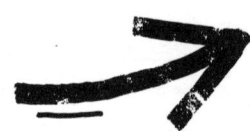

Deep Sleep is where our body does its best 'fixing' – growing, healing, and getting stronger. Your brain is less busy, but this stage helps you remember things and feel rested when you wake up. It's also when your immune system gets a boost.

REM (Rapid Eye Movement) sleep is the part of sleep when our brains are most active and when we are most likely to dream. It gets its name because our eyes flicker behind our closed eyelids when it happens. In childhood, REM sleep is particularly important for helping young brains to develop.

Long story short – a LOT of important work happens while you sleep, particularly at your age, and getting plenty of it is key to your happiness and health.

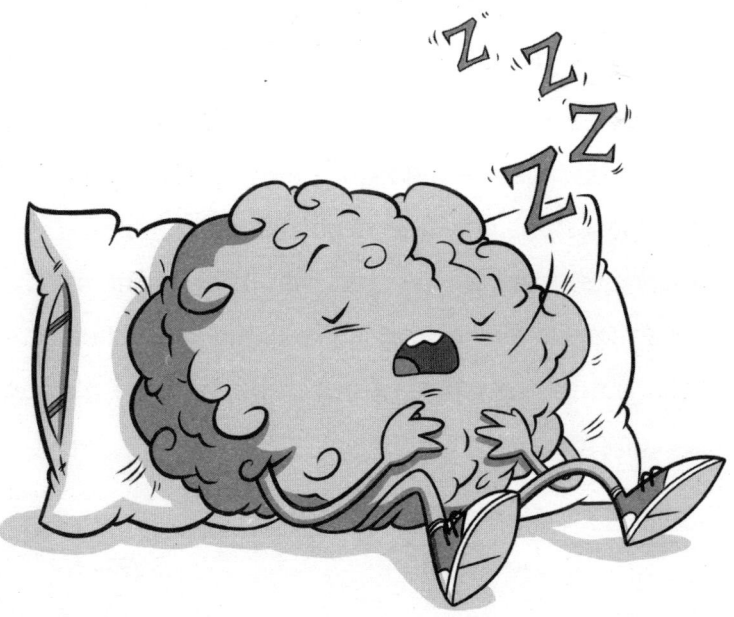

Our emotions and experiences can be processed and short-term memories are transferred into our long-term memory bank. I like to picture my brain as a filing cabinet, with any new experiences from the day being stored away in the right section while I sleep.

So, establishing a good bedtime routine is one of the kindest things we can do for ourselves. Look at babies and toddlers. When we're very young, our parents will guide us through a bedtime routine – if you have younger siblings, you might see this going on at home. It might involve bathtime, story time, milk and a cuddle before being rocked to sleep. If the routine is disrupted – on holiday, for example – a baby might wake up more than usual.

This doesn't change as you get older: your quality of sleep also relies on a good bedtime routine. What may change is that now *you* might be responsible for the routine instead of your parents. They might still be involved with elements of it, like giving you a goodnight kiss, but on the whole, it's over to you to go through the process.

FUTURE YOU

While you're still living at home, you may have other people around, helping you with bedtime and reminding you to brush your teeth or go up to bed at a certain time. But as we grow up, it's good to become more independent when we can. So getting into a great routine now will help us with tackling these tasks with few reminders, even if we might still need help to complete them.

Ideally you'll begin your routine at roughly the same time every evening – around an hour before bed – then work through the same steps. The familiarity will train your brain to start feeling tired at that time.

Here's an idea of how your bedtime routine could look, but you can design this in a way that works for you.

 Pick a time to go to bed – for example, 8 p.m.

 At 7 p.m., turn off your screens. If you have a smartphone, leave it downstairs or put it in a drawer.

Our brain releases a hormone called **melatonin** that regulates our sleep. In the evening, our melatonin levels naturally rise, telling our body it's time to go to sleep. Our melatonin levels then go back to normal in the day.

If we're not careful though, our melatonin production can be disrupted, leading to problems sleeping. The blue light emitted from smartphones, tablets, TVs and computers confuses the brain into thinking it's daytime, waking us up again when we should be winding down. This is why putting our devices away is key for a healthy bedtime.

Additionally, some types of content — like loud, violent movies or video games — can work against our sleep too.

★ Drink a small glass of water. It's important to stay hydrated while we sleep.

★ Bathroom time. Brush your teeth and wash your face.

★ Have a shower or bath if you want one.

★ Get into your PJs – aah, cosy time!

★ Put your day's clothes in the laundry basket unless you're wearing some of them again tomorrow and give your room a quick tidy.

★ If there's anything you need to prepare for the next day, do so – but be mindful to do it calmly. Rushing around sends our brain the message that we're still active and not ready for sleep, so mindfully slow down your body movements, whatever you're doing.

A really important part of our bedtime routine is finding something enjoyable and relaxing to do. Here are some ideas of things to do that *also* make us feel restful and sleepy:

Reading. Reading is a really enriching process for your mind. Studies have shown that just a few minutes of reading can reduce your stress levels and maybe even help you live longer when done regularly. Pick any book, magazine or comic you enjoy, or listen to an audiobook – there are no rules here!

Journalling. Writing in a diary is a brilliant way of unwinding. It also gives us a chance to look back on our day and think about what went well. Even better, try to focus on three things that you have been grateful for today.

Having a bedtime chat with someone in your family. Quietly talking through the events of your day or any worries you have, can have a lovely calming effect before bed.

Cuddling your pet if you have one. Stroking a furry friend brings down your blood pressure and is a very soothing end to the day. (As long as your dog doesn't demand walkies!)

Switch off the light and go to sleep!

TOP TIP

If you've spent time on your bed during the day, playing or eating or doing homework, your brain might associate it with those activities rather than resting.

So try to keep your bed for sleeping only, and you'll be more likely to nod off when you get under the covers. Plus, less chance of crumbs in your sheets. Sweet dreams!

DR ALEX'S MORNING ROUTINE

Over the years, I've found my perfect morning routine. It works well for me so I don't really change it, which is great because it means I have a pretty solid structure that saves me from thinking about what I have to do each morning.

I wake up at 6.30 a.m., have a drink of water, make my bed, brush my teeth and shower. Then I have a hot drink, do ten minutes of meditation to clear my mind, take my dog outside for a walk, have breakfast and get ready to start my work at 9 a.m.

Adding together these happy habits at the start of my day makes me feel positive and alert, with boosted dopamine levels. Best of all, I feel grounded from the benefits of movement and nature.

Whenever I need to adjust this routine (say I'm travelling or staying with a friend), I try to keep as many elements in there as I can. But it's never quite the same, and it's always a nice feeling to come home and get back to the structure that helps me thrive.

BEDROOM BASICS

Tidying your room may sound like a boring chore, or even punishment, forced on you by your parents. It can feel like hard work and as though there's a million things you'd rather be doing. So, let's focus on what's *good* about tidying.

Studies have shown that **clean bedrooms are good for our minds.** The act of tidying your room can itself be an act of self-nurture – a mindful activity that peacefully brings you into the moment and helps you gain control of your surroundings. If you really struggle to get the motivation, there are hacks to make cleaning more enjoyable:

★ Time it. Set a timer to see how quickly you can get your room **SPOTLESS**. This makes it into a game, and you can try and beat your best score every time.

★ Connect it to something you like. Maybe you enjoy listening to music or watching streamers on YouTube. Play the tunes or videos *while* you clean, so that something you enjoy combines with your happy habit to get more done.

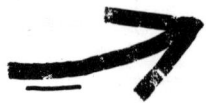

MAKE YOUR BED

Let's start with an obvious one. I remember thinking, *what's the big deal with making my bed? I'm just going to mess it up again later when I get back into it at bedtime!*

But it turns out there is something strangely rewarding about coming home to a neat bed. Admiral McRaven (that is a pretty cool name), a now-retired commander in the US Navy, mentioned the importance of making your bed in a talk, which you can find on YouTube. In it, he said:

> If by chance you have a miserable day, you will come home to a bed that is made – that *you* made – and a made bed gives you encouragement that tomorrow will be better. If you want to change the world, start off by making your bed.

Yes, that's right – a top military leader took time out to talk about fluffing pillows and folding sheets. Being a soldier doesn't mean forgetting about things like tidying; it actually makes it even more important. **Doing your best means taking care of the small things and making an effort to prepare well each day.**

Scientifically, it makes sense. Dopamine, the reward hormone, is released in our brain every time we tick off this kind of task. This makes us feel good and optimistic that we can achieve whatever else there is to do that day.

So, take **30 seconds** to make your bed and give yourself a little win at the start of the day!

GIVE YOUR ROOM A QUICK ONCE-OVER

Giving your room a quick tidy before school can leave you feeling calmer and less stressed. You are less likely to lose items if they are put away regularly – or injure yourself tripping over them!

A few minutes of tidying every day also means that you are less likely to have to do a massive clean-up during your precious weekend time. So put away those PJs, slam-dunk yesterday's clothes into the laundry basket and take down any plates or cups to the kitchen and wash them up. Future (weekend) you will be grateful they don't have to carry a week's worth in one go!

GET DRESSED AND PACK YOUR SCHOOLBAG

Take a few minutes to gather the items you need for the day ahead. This means you are less likely to forget anything important and have a last-minute panic. A printed-out list of things to remember and actions you need to take can also help you stay on task.

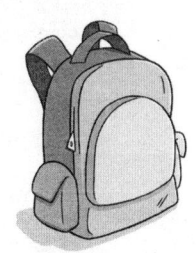

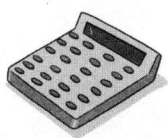

The items might include your uniform, a filled-up water bottle, textbooks, your pencil case, a change of clothes or any items needed for an after-school club.

Make sure you also take out anything from your bag that needs putting away, chucking away (yesterday's banana peel) or washing.

Once you have everything, get dressed and pack your bag. You're done!

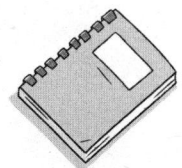

You may prefer to lay out your uniform and pack your bag before bed. This is a great idea because it makes mornings feel that bit calmer. In fact, our brains are more prone to feel stress or worry in the first hour of waking up, because of a stress hormone called **cortisol**.

So, anything we can do at night that makes mornings feel less stressful is *extra* useful.

Remember though, there will be some days when, for any number of reasons, we feel low on energy or not up to carrying out all our daily tasks. That's fine, and normal – human beings aren't meant to be perfect all the time. Building these habits over time will enhance your overall well-being, but it's OK to skip a day or two when you need to, and you won't ruin the habit as long as you're doing it most days.

HABIT HACK: MAKE GOOD HABITS OBVIOUS

You've probably noticed how the most *unhealthy* things have the *brightest* packaging. This is because companies know they have to get your attention to make you want things that are bad for you.

Think about it. Fast-food restaurants have massive bright signs and sweets are in luminous packaging right beside the checkout, whereas things like broccoli are just . . . well . . . broccoli.

Poor broccoli. It is a beautiful thing, but it doesn't have a team of people working behind the scenes to make people notice it. Well, I'm making it my job to **MAKE BROCCOLI NOTICEABLE AGAIN**.

OK, so maybe that's a bit much, but we should remember that although there are people trying to make unhealthy things noticeable, we should try and notice healthy ones too.

Happy, healthy habits are not always **easy** and not always **obvious**. So we have to make them easy and obvious!

The places where you spend most of your time, such as your bedroom and the kitchen, are like a *playground* for your brain. It is scanning the area, noticing things like an excitable puppy who bounces around sniffing everything and everyone.

What we have to do is **make the good things easy to notice, and the less good things harder**. Maybe you want to play fewer video games, so you put your controller in a drawer, not out where you can see it and get tempted.

Hide your crisps in the tallest, darkest cupboard and put the apples out on the table with a sign saying **EAT ME**. (Though we all have the odd day where we still eat the crisps too, and that's OK!)

Leave a banana on top of the TV remote to remind you to have fruit before you watch any telly. It will seem strange for a while, but people will get used to it.

CREATE SIGNS (OR CUES)

So, we should set up our living spaces to send messages to our brain. This means leaving out cues, or clues, that direct us towards healthy habits.

Have you ever noticed that when you go into the kitchen, you start to feel hungry for a snack, even though you weren't before? That's because it's where you usually eat, and you have a *cue* that tells your brain you must be hungry.

Or maybe you don't feel like doing homework, but once you sit at your tidy desk, it becomes easier. This is because **the places we are in can *remind* us to do certain things and even *encourage* us.**

So we should make our bedroom a place that reminds us to . . . can you guess what the answer is?

That's right – **PARTY!**

No, not really! The answer is sleep. Go to bed. **ZZZZZ**.

We need a room that gives us cues to be sleepy. So let's think about that. How can we design our room in a way that makes us sleepy?

LIGHTS

Create cues with the lights in your room. Gradually lower the brightness of the lights as you get towards bedtime. This makes our brain really feel like it is becoming night and want to sleep.

RELAXATION

Put your book out on your pillow where you can see it, because reading is a great bedtime habit. That will remind you to read before bed and put you into your sleepy routine.

PYJAMAS OR NIGHTIE

Lay them out on the bed and change into them at the same time every night. Just like a football kit can put you in a sporty mood, or a cape can make you feel like a superhero (I haven't tried that. . .), PJs can make you feel like sleeping. Or make you feel like a *very tired* superhero, pyjama-girl or ZZZman, saving the world from late nights . . .

But remember, it works the opposite way too. So try not to have things in your room that might tempt you to stay up. Video-game consoles, PCs with blue lights and mobile phones all keep our brain awake, so we don't even want them to be visible in our rooms. If they are out of sight, they'll be easier to avoid.

All of our habits benefit from the way we design and organize our environment. **The spaces we create can lead us towards healthy or unhappy habits,** so it is up to us to create encouraging, happy spaces.

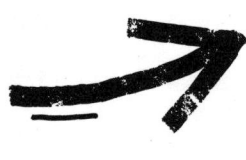

Think of your life and your home a bit like a video game. In a game, we often know which way we are supposed to go and what we are supposed to do without the game *actually* telling us. This is called 'choice architecture'. Maybe they create a clear path in one direction or have a floating gem you can see in the distance. Whatever it is, they design the environment to encourage you in a certain direction.

So think of yourself like a video-game designer – only instead of points or levels, you have happy habits, and you want to design your maps (rooms) in a way that takes you towards them. It might mean hiding your mobile phone under the bed or putting your TV control in a bowl of oranges, but it will encourage you to make happier choices.

And at the end of a long day of good choices, there is nothing better than a good, long sleep.

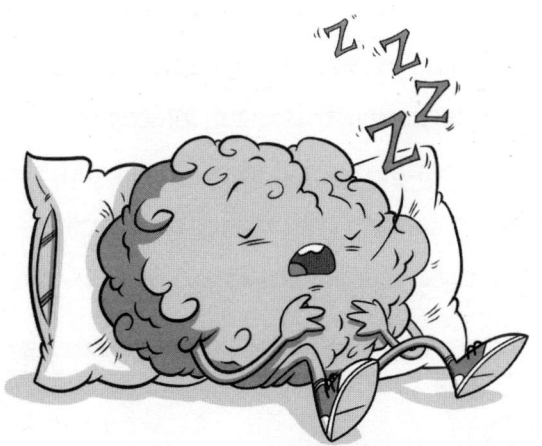

HAPPY HABIT 6: LET'S TALK ABOUT SCREEN TIME

You may have noticed that I spoke quite a bit about games consoles, mobile phones and computer screens in the section on sleep. That is because these electronic devices energize our brains in a way that makes sleeping difficult, so we have to be careful not to use them around bedtime.

In fact, we need to be careful about our screen time *all the time.*

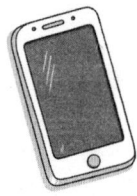 You were born into a world brimming with screens, from smartphones and tablets to TVs and games consoles. Schoolwork, TV shows, YouTube, movies and video games are just some of the things we can access via screens, and who knows what's to come in the future. There is so much brilliant information 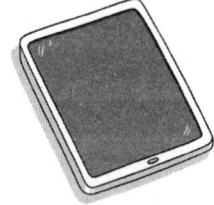 and entertainment at our fingertips, along with endless ways to connect with friends and family when we can't see them in person.

There are countless devices, too, from TVs to gaming consoles to laptops, tablets and phones. Perhaps you have a smartphone already, or are begging your parents to let you have one. Most likely the content you can access if you do have your own phone is carefully monitored by your parent or caregiver.

In an ideal world, my advice as a doctor would be that young people should leave smartphones alone for as long as possible. I would suggest no smartphones before age fourteen and no social media before age sixteen. There will be plenty of time to make use of them as an adult, and childhood is a really precious time when real-life adventures and interactions with others are much better for your developing brain than spending too much time on a screen.

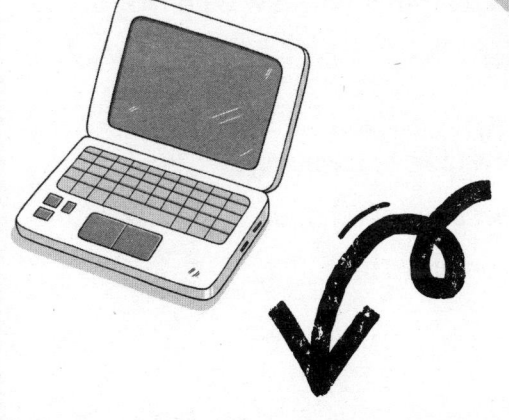

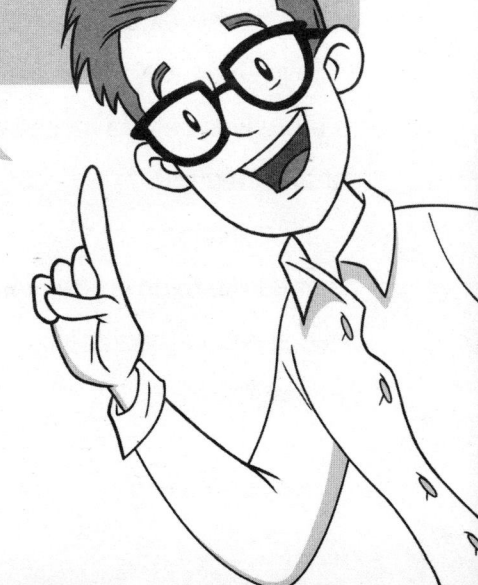

But I'm not here to ban screen time. Realistically, our world makes it very hard to avoid screens completely, and when it comes to things like smartphones and social media, you and your family will probably be having regular discussions about what feels appropriate for you – and that's as it should be. It's also worth just saying that for some people with physical disabilities or neurodivergence diagnoses, screens and apps help them access the world around them in ways they may not be able to otherwise, and that's OK.

Studies have shown that usually, human willpower alone isn't enough to break a phone addiction – because they really are SO addictive. Installing an app that limits your screen time can be a helpful tool, and many adults I know, including me, rely on this.

When I became old enough to have a phone, it was a Nokia 3310, which had a very simple digital screen. It took ages to type out a text, and the fanciest game was something called *Snake*! I feel lucky in some ways because I couldn't get stuck on it for too long, as there was only so much I could do with it. There was nothing to get addicted to.

What I'd like to do is offer you a few tools to encourage general good habits with screens – whichever devices you have. It's all a question of balance.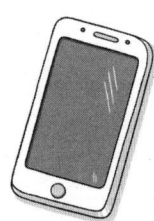

IT'S NOT JUST YOU!

Firstly, it's important to bear in mind that things like computer games and social media are designed to be addictive. Remember we spoke about how we can create cravings for ourselves and how 'choice architecture' leads us towards certain habits? Well, the people who design technology and online platforms know **THE MOST** about this and programme their designs to attract us and keep us scrolling.

So it's no surprise that many of us do feel addicted from time to time – our brains are responding to something that has been specifically created to keep us wanting more! Adults struggle with it too, so finding a good balance now will help you in the future, as we adjust the devices we're on as we get older, join the workplace and new technology becomes available.

Don't feel guilty for bingeing half a dozen YouTube videos or getting carried away playing *Fortnite* – we all do it occasionally! But at the same time, remember that you are in control, and if you feel like you're spending too much time watching or playing something, you have the power to step away from it. You can always come back to it later.

It's usually the case that we get most enjoyment at the beginning of watching or playing something, then we start to enjoy it less the more time goes on – yet our instinct is often to keep doing it. So, we have to create our own reminders to take breaks. When you play a game or have some screen time, **set an alarm for thirty minutes**. When the alarm goes off, stop and take a break – maybe do some star jumps, head outside with some paper and pencils or anything else that breaks you out of video-game/ YouTube zombie mode. This will give you a chance to think about how much time you have spent online and encourage you to make a choice about other, happier ways to spend the next thirty minutes.

That small break (or long one if you do a million star jumps) allows you to consider doing something else, but mostly it allows you to *think*. Often when we are online, **we lose track of time.** If we regain a sense of it by taking breaks, we can at least be aware of how much time we are spending.

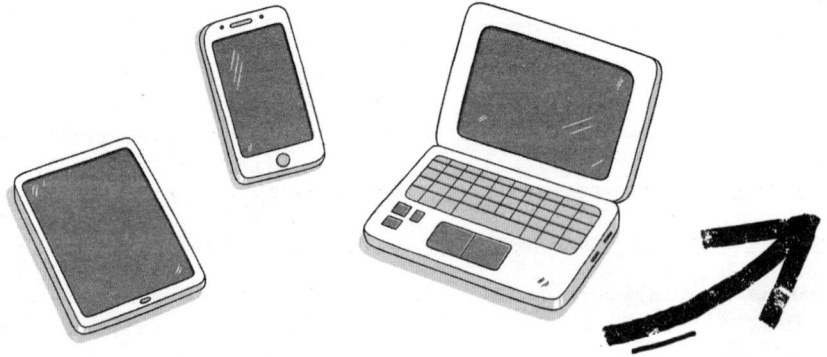

INFORMATION DIET

Just like the food on our plates, our 'information diet' can be good or bad. What we choose to watch – or 'consume' – has a huge effect on us and our mood. So it's a good idea to ask yourself, as you're looking at something online or watching TV, **is this making me feel happy and engaged?** Am I learning something, or laughing my socks off? Or is it making me sad or bored? Am I comparing myself negatively to someone on the screen in front of me?

Don't hesitate to step away from something if you figure out that it's not making you feel good. We all react to things in different ways, so what your friend enjoys watching may not be as enjoyable for you. Finding the perfect show that always gives you a feel-good boost, on the other hand, is an amazing part of modern life!

Growing up, I loved David Attenborough's *Planet Earth* and *Blue Planet* documentaries, and I still enjoy them because they remind me that the world is really big and full of beautiful places, landscapes and animals. They take me on a little holiday away from anything stressful that might be on my mind and help me 'zoom out' from my own problems.

Perhaps baking shows or *Match of the Day* have the same effect on you?

Your tastes will change with time, so **keep exploring what's out there** (as long as it's safe and age-appropriate), and don't confine yourself to just one thing – especially if it's not making you happy.

SCREENTIME VS REAL-LIFE CONNECTION

Humans are designed to be social creatures who regularly spend time with other people. We get a wonderful sense of belonging and purpose when we're around friends, family and school or workmates. These relationships are essential for our well-being – science shows that people who regularly spend time surrounded by others tend to be healthier and live longer.

So while screen time can be fun, so is meeting up with your friends. Or, of course, it can be a mix of both – who doesn't love hanging out with friends, eating food and watching a Netflix movie?

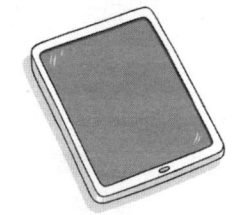

But don't forget to make time for proper face-to-face time too – whether it's walking to school with your brother or sister, a game of rounders in the park or heading out on an adventure at the weekend. **Nothing is better for your health and happiness than human connection.**

FAMILY PHONE LOCK-UP

Some families have a great joint habit that involves everyone putting their phone into an 'unplug box' at the same time. This encourages family members to disconnect from their devices and reconnect with each other for special moments like mealtimes or board-game nights.

You can even add a reward element for everyone to enjoy if they leave the phones in the box for the allotted time – for example, if everyone puts their phones away for dinner every night for a month, you've earned a family trip to the cinema!

Suggest this to your parents – say that **you** will have no screens after 6 p.m. (for example) if **they** have no screens either.

FIRST AND LAST HOUR OF THE DAY

This is probably the most important habit I'd advise everyone to stick to – including myself. I think it's manageable for everyone (albeit with a little practice!).

The habit is: **avoid screens for the first hour of the day after you wake up, and the last hour before you go to sleep.** This is really important to our brain health. We need to allow our brain some time and space to wake naturally from our sleeping state, and the blue light of a phone screen can interrupt this process. This in turn can lead to us feeling anxious and stressed – not the best way to start your day.

If your smartphone is also your alarm, try buying an alarm clock and putting your phone away in a drawer so that you aren't tempted to look at it as soon as you open your eyes.

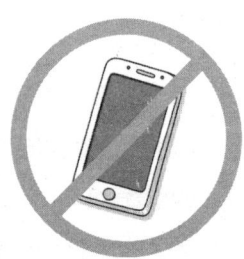

For similar reasons, it's important to wind down our brains properly at the end of the day – so steering clear of the screens at least an hour before bed is a brilliant habit to get into. Stick that phone in the drawer after tea and forget about it! Then, do something like relaxing with a good book instead of scrolling.

DIGITAL DETOX

Bear with me on this one, but from a scientific point of view, steering clear of all screens for a whole day – or longer – is like a five-star holiday for our brains. It may sound rubbish – not to mention hard – but hear me out. It's one of the best things we can do for our well-being.

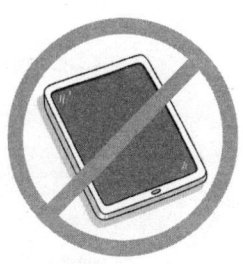

The benefits are huge. **The longer you are off your devices, the better you will be able to focus on one thing at a time.** You will think more clearly, and your mind will be less likely to spiral into anxious thoughts. You are likely to have more meaningful and rewarding conversations with the people around you, and you'll enjoy the calm feeling of living in the moment.

It may feel tricky and uncomfortable at first, but stick with it. It's so good for your health to do this from time to time that it's worth it!

During a digital detox, why not plan lots of alternative activities to keep you on track – make your favourite meal, play some football, visit your friend or go for a stomp in the woods!

I really don't want to get into the habit of checking my work emails and messages late at night – that's no fun! So the more you can develop good habits around screens now, the easier we will find it to **SWITCH OFF OUR DEVICES** and enjoy our free time as an adult. (Even if we have a busy job and lots of people messaging us all the time!)

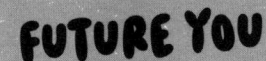

FUTURE YOU

As a final thought on this habit, here's a statistic I found recently:

The average British person spends five hours a day looking at a phone screen.

If they did this every day from ages eighteen to seventy-eight they would spend . . . wait for it . . . **over twelve years of their adult life looking at a phone**. That's waking hours only – so twelve years of entire days. Think how much you could do with that block of time if it was completely freed up. Or even just half of it. Imagine all the books you could read, places you could explore, cakes you could bake, new languages or sports you could learn. You could teach yourself to play the guitar, the piano, the drums . . . the possibilities are amazing. It's up to us how we spend our precious free time, so let's think carefully about how much of it we want to give to our devices.

PART 4: PLAN

HAPPY HABIT 7: HOMEWORK AND EXAM PREP

You might look at the title of this chapter and feel tempted to fast-forward past it . . . believe me, I totally get that feeling!

As someone who left my AS level chemistry revision until two days before the exam (and got a D because of it), I know homework and exams can feel quite boring or stressful, or be something we'd rather not think about all.

The annoying thing is that schoolwork is an essential part of life. There's no avoiding it, and trying to put it off only makes it harder. So let's try and figure out the easiest, happiest approach to doing the work we have to do.

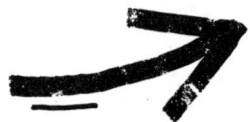

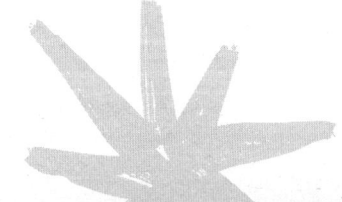

The good news is that by working towards a target in the right way, you can shine brightly while keeping your stress levels low. Perfect grades aren't the main goal here – **it's about being prepared, doing the best you can and staying happy and healthy in the process.**

Everyone has different learning styles. Those who like to do their schoolwork the second it's been set; those who are desperately trying to finish it at breakfast on the day that it's due; and everyone in between. Where do you think you fit on that scale?

I work best under pressure, but I don't like being anxious, so at school I had to find a middle ground where I wasn't leaving my revision until the last moment (as that would make me anxious), but I genuinely found it hard to get started until the day of the exam was looming near on the calendar.

At medical school there were people who sat around working all day long. They always had their books out, even in the cafeteria at lunchtime or at a quiz night in the pub. Sometimes I thought I should do that too. But what I noticed was that they didn't always get the best grades. It really baffled me at first – perhaps they were going through the motions of working, but because they never switched off or rested, they didn't end up doing as

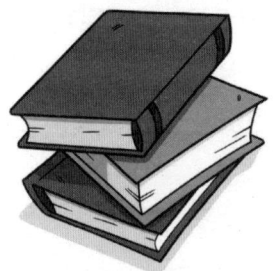 well as they might have done. I realized that the people who got the best grades tended to have good social lives and join in with sports or clubs, as well as working hard.

A healthy habit here is to be either 'on' work mode or 'off' it. Try not to mix the two. Twenty minutes of focused study in a quiet place will be far more productive than two hours of half-heartedly looking at your notes while chatting to your friends or scrolling on your phone.

And planning your time clearly will make all the difference. When we decide on a certain time to work, we regain all the time before (when we might be worrying about when we will get our work done) and all the time afterwards, when we feel free because we have nothing left to do.

GAMIFY YOUR LEARNING

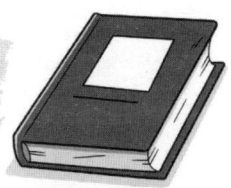

By turning learning into a game, we can create rewards and get stuff done effectively and on time. Rather than treating your history revision as a big scary mountain of dates that you're convinced you will never cram into your brain (again, I've been there!), set yourself a time challenge and promise yourself a reward at the end of it.

Start by setting a timer for yourself – for example, set a twenty-minute timer and give the task your full concentration during that time.

When the timer goes off, take two minutes to look over your work and recite to yourself what you've learned, as this teaches your brain to retain the information.

Then unleash your reward! Choose something fun just for you, whether it's time on your game console or curling up with a chapter of your new book.

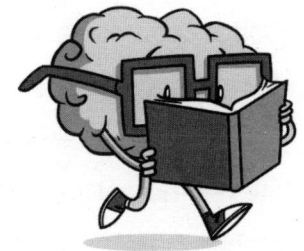

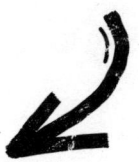

During exam season at uni, my housemates and I would revise in our rooms for an hour, then meet in the kitchen for a chat and a cup of tea.

BELIEVE IN YOURSELF

At school, I had undiagnosed **ADHD** and found starting tasks very daunting. Concentrating was difficult too. I used to worry I was lazy, but I was wrong. It had nothing to do with laziness; it was my ADHD. I would put off my homework for as long as possible because I was worried about not getting the best grades and letting myself down. It felt easier not to start a task at all rather than begin it with the fear of getting it wrong.

Luckily, I had an amazing teacher in secondary school – Mr Harris, my history teacher – who helped change my outlook. He was very funny, a huge character, who taught through storytelling. He was good at spotting people who had potential but needed a little boost of encouragement.

One day he pulled me aside and said he could tell I was lacking self-belief. He encouraged me to enjoy history and have fun, to find my groove without overthinking it.

ADHD, or **Attention Deficit Hyperactivity Disorder**, is a condition that describes how some people have different attention spans. People with ADHD sometimes find it hard to sit still for long periods, or wait to do things that excite us. Because of this, people with ADHD can get distracted easily (by things we find more interesting), forget things, or have trouble remembering rules at home or school. Adults often have to change how they do things to help children with ADHD and understand the different ways they think, like trying new routines, using exercise, or eating healthy foods. Not everything works the same for every child, though, so teachers and parents sometimes have to try different ideas to see what helps.

If you too have a neurodivergence diagnosis, my personal experience is that while my day-to-day life has been massively helped by the habits in this book, also make sure you speak to a teacher or caregiver if you need additional support.

His faith in me changed everything. Just like a talented football pro can't play well if they have no self-belief, a bright kid can't get good grades if they're convinced they are a failure.

I hope you'll have the same luck I did and have teachers like Mr Harris – there are plenty of them out there. But whatever happens, and no matter what anyone else says or doesn't say, back yourself. **You're worth it**.

HOMEWORK: JUST START

As you get older, homework starts to play a bigger role in your education. Getting it done on time, and to the best of your ability, can sometimes feel overwhelming. There might be one or two subjects that you find particularly challenging, or where you don't get amazing grades even when you try your hardest, so it all feels a bit pointless.

This can make us feel like we don't even want to start. But if we delay our homework and make up loads of excuses, the homework doesn't go away. Our teacher will still expect us to do it, even if we get an extension and hand it in late.

The longer we put it off, the more miserable we make ourselves, as our worrying about it will just increase.

So my top tip is simple: **just start it.**

Have you ever jumped into a cold swimming pool? Dipping your toe in and thinking about how cold it is going to be is always unbearable. You spend all the time thinking about how bad the experience will be, but then you do it and it feels fine. The key is to **make the leap**, then you free yourself of all the time worrying about what it will be like. Homework is the same: worrying about doing it or putting it off is *genuinely worse* than actually doing it. So get started.

As soon as you get going, those anxieties will start to fade, and the task will start to feel more possible. Even though the water might feel cold, you'll feel better for having dunked.

Mel Robbins, bestselling author and motivational speaker, has a brilliant '5-second rule' that may help when it comes to starting your homework – and anything else that you're feeling reluctant to do but that you have to get done.

It involves counting down from **5 to 1** – like a rocket about to launch into space.

Step 1: The thought.

'I should start my homework.'

Step 2: The countdown.

5...4...3...2...1

(You can do it in a big, American announcer voice if you like.)

Step 3: Blast off! Follow through and start the task immediately.

Why does this work? Well, Mel realized that if your brain focuses on the countdown, it won't distract itself by coming up with reasons not to do the 'thing'.

Once you eliminate all those thoughts and distractions by concentrating on **5, 4, 3, 2, 1**, you will feel prepared to start.

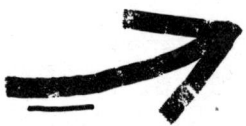

HABIT HACK: THE TWO-MINUTE TRY

If something feels hard and you don't want to start, just do the first tiny part that takes two minutes or less.

For example: want to read a book? Just read one page.

Want to clean your room? Just pick up one thing.

Want to practise piano? Just sit down and play for two minutes.

Once you start, it's often easier to keep going. Your brain gets a little boost of **dopamine** (the reward hormone) for getting the first part done, and often this is enough to keep us going.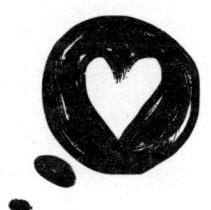

But even if you stop after two minutes, you're still building the habit!

It's like **Tricking your brain** to get started by making it super small and easy.

BUT WHERE? HOW? WHEN?

➡️ Before putting the 'just start' or 'two-minute try' rule into action with your homework, make sure you've set yourself up in a helpful environment. Remember, your environment can *encourage* you.

➡️ Choose a quiet place where you can work without distractions, with a clear area to spread out your stuff. This might be the kitchen table or a desk in your bedroom.

➡️ Try to keep this as your homework place without moving around each time – this will send a message to your brain as soon as you sit down that it's time to work.

➡️ Having said that, a practice called body doubling can also help you stay on track, especially if you have a neurodivergence diagnosis. This is where someone else is physically in the same space as you while you work, but they are doing their own thing. It might look like you doing your homework in the kitchen while your grown-up prepares a meal or sorts the dirty washing.

➡ In the same way, if you can find a similar time of day to work (maybe before or after dinner), your mind will get into the groove of that routine. Again, it will feel easier to do it just because you've done it at the same time every day this week.

➡ Make a plan. Figure out what homework you're going to do on which day, and make sure you have the right books and equipment before you start each homework session. All set? Off you go!

Looking back, I wish I could tell kid Alex to do his homework instead of putting it off and anxiously stewing over the thought of it. I could have just set a twenty-minute timer, done my best, then run off with my friends for a game of footie and forgotten all about it.

That reminds me . . .

DON'T FORGET TO COLLECT YOUR REWARD

This is a big one. You don't just have to have rewards when you stick to a habit for a long time – **it's actually *good* to reward yourself every time.** So promise yourself a little reward at the end of your homework – whether it's a hot chocolate, hanging out with a friend or reading a chapter of your favourite graphic novel. You earned it!

And by associating something pleasurable with something tough, your brain will be more up for the homework challenge (because after a couple of days, it will know that the reward is coming!).

IF YOU GET STUCK, NO PROBLEM!

Homework is there to reveal what we don't know, as well as what we DO know. So, if you get stuck, ask for help from a grown-up or a trusted friend. Everyone has to do this from time to time, and it's how we learn.

WHY EXAMS CAN FEEL SCARY ... BUT DON'T HAVE TO

Tests and exams can feel like the last things you want to make into a habit. Unfortunately, before the age of eighteen you will have to do *hundreds* of tests, so the question is, how can we create habits that make tests less stressful?

How can we shift our mindset to see tests as nothing more than an opportunity to revise our knowledge, do our best and learn how we need to improve?

Well, the first step is to ask that question. If you realize that tests are just a part of life and you want to work out how to make them more manageable, then you are *already* starting a great habit. The happy habit of *perspective*.

So accept tests. Prepare for tests. **And do your best. That is all there is to do.**

In terms of what you shouldn't do: try not to worry about them, because it genuinely doesn't help, and life is too great a thing to be spent worrying about tests.

Try to see that **you are more than your test results**. A high score doesn't make you a better person, and a lower one doesn't make you worse. It reflects how much correct information you were able to write down on that piece of paper on that day.

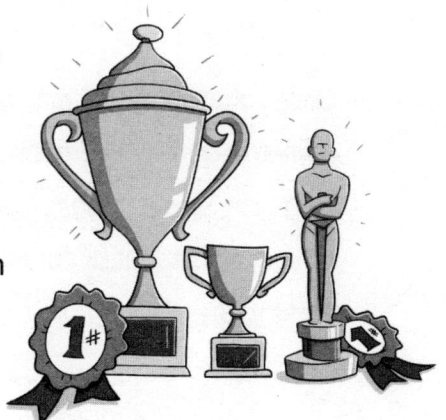

Remember that people – your teachers and your family – may want you to do well but they are not demanding that you do *everything*. All you can do is your best, so doing your best is *all* you have to focus on.

They will also not change their opinion of you because you either do well on a test or receive a lower mark. All anyone can judge is your effort, and the only person who *really knows* the effort you have put in is you. But please never suffer in silence. If you are struggling at school, please talk to a trusted grown-up like a teacher, support worker, or a parent or guardian and just let them know you are finding things tough. They will be able to support you.

So, try to turn this idea into a habit: **The only opinion That matters is my own, and all I ask is That I try.**

Occasionally, there are exams that do have a bearing on something else, like getting into a certain school or university. Here, the same things count – your effort and your own opinion of your effort, but of course, your performance has an impact on what you are then able to do. Usually, we have the opportunity to try again if things don't go to plan, so remember it is never the end of the world.

But also remember that *even if* you don't get to try again, and some opportunity is missed because of a test mark, that is fine too. We all miss out sometimes – we learn, and we get better. Some of the most successful people in the world failed tests or didn't get into university. In fact, many of them only became successful *because* they failed a test and focused on something else that they realized they were good at.

So remember, if you don't feel like you are good at tests, **find lots of other things that you *do* feel good at.** Someone great at tests may not be able to draw like you or run as far; they might not be a great listener like you are or as funny as you are. There are many *thousands* of ways to be capable in this world, and if a particular test doesn't test the way in which you are capable, then believe you can find one that does.

Whatever happens, I'll say it again: do your best. Do your best to revise, do your best to stay calm and do your best in the exam itself. Then you can feel confident that you did everything you could.

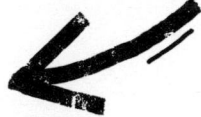

And as you are going into that exam hall, tell yourself,

I've done my best. I couldn't have prepared any better.

And as you open the paper, say,

You've got this, buddy.

It might sound silly at first, but speaking to yourself like a supportive friend when you face a challenge on your own, is *a great habit*.

TOP TIP

As humans, we tend to overestimate the challenge and underestimate our ability to handle it. Bear this in mind when prepping for an exam. You've got this!

One day, you'll look back and see the exams weren't as bad as you maybe thought they were when you were living them.
They aren't the be-all and end-all, just a part of life.

DON'T LET GO OF OTHER THINGS

At times, when I was revising for school or medical exams, my sleep routine would go out of the window. I'd stay up late, eat junk food, stop exercising and avoid seeing my friends. I was convinced that if I put everything into preparing for the next exam, nothing else mattered. Surely being permanently surrounded by my laptop, books and papers was the best way to cram in those facts?!

But come the day of the exam, I would feel tired and frazzled. I realize now that all the things I had let go of, like a fun kickaround with my friends, were things that would have helped me deal with the stress.

Good sleep, good nutrition, movement and social interaction all help our brain to function well. They blitz the clouds of anxiety that may build around exam time by taking us out of our minds and into our bodies.

So whatever you do, make sure to schedule in some fun and relaxation, and plenty of nourishing meals among the revision.

TOP TIP

As for the actual revision – **you've got this**.

Follow the homework tips in this chapter to make sure you're working in a calm, organized environment.

Test yourself regularly – you could ask a friend or family member to quiz you.

Allow yourself plenty of time with each subject, so that if you struggle with a topic while revising, you have enough time to ask for help and work through it at a slower pace.

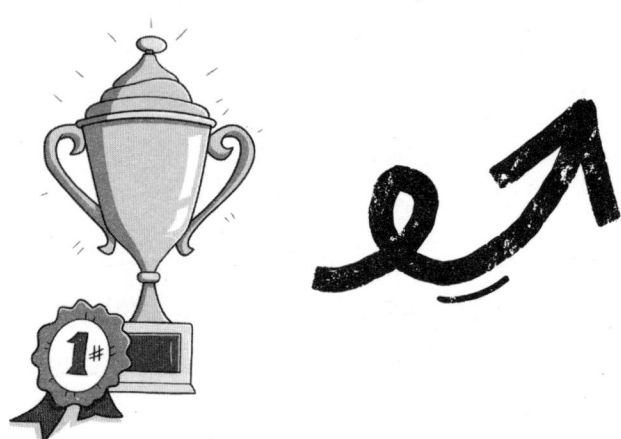

THE NIGHT BEFORE . . . AND EXAM DAY

Do everything you can to get a good night's rest the night before your exam. This is more important than trying to do last-minute revision.

Reassure yourself that you've prepared, and make a conscious decision not to worry what will happen on the day – that is out of your control now.

So here's an example of a happy, healthy night before an exam.

An hour and a half before bed, decide to finish revision, because relaxing is *important* work too. Tell your family that you'll help them with the dinner because it's nice to take your mind off your work.

Help lay the table and enjoy the meal, which might contain chicken, greens or butternut squash (because they contain **tryptophan**, which helps us sleep) and then all eat together. Sometimes exams can make us feel quite alone, so a meal with other people can make us feel better. Just make sure you don't talk about exams!

Finish off with a banana (more tryptophan), then a warm bath and thirty minutes of reading a book. Soon you should start to feel tired, and then you can do the best revision possible, which happens in your sleep.

I mean that: *in your sleep.* When you have spent time learning any new thing, a good sleep provides a chance for your brain to 'consolidate it', which means turning it from *learning* into *knowledge.* So remember that your **sleep is part of your revision and preparation process.**

On the day itself, a good sleep will have you feeling rested. Try to have a good breakfast (porridge is great for slow-release energy) and a glass of water.

Then make sure you turn up to the exam hall in plenty of time, so you're not feeling rushed.

Then all that's left to do is your best!

AFTER THE EXAM

It's tempting to compare notes with your friends as soon as you walk out of the exam hall. You know the kind of thing –

> Phew! That wasn't as bad as I thought.

or

> What did you put for the second question?

or

> Arghhh, I ran out of time . . . I've definitely failed.

Just make sure the conversations don't stress you out. You may realize that it's better for your mental well-being not to discuss the exams afterwards – it certainly was for me. I would sometimes hear what other people had put for a certain question, assume that they were right and that my answer was wrong, and miserably conclude that I'd failed the exam. . . then later on find out I'd done OK.

DEALING WITH FAILURE

Sometimes we don't get the results we were hoping for. It's a rubbish feeling, especially if we put our time and energy into preparing for the exam. Or even if we didn't! Nobody enjoys failure, but you can learn to live with it. And even better, you can learn from it.

Have you ever heard the saying, **'Failure is data'**? It's the idea that when we fail at something, it helps us figure out where the gaps in our knowledge are. It's not something to be embarrassed about, it's just data – information, so that we can know how to avoid the gaps next time.

I know all about failure. The first time I applied to medical school, I didn't manage to get the grades I needed. It was an awful feeling at the time, and I thought that my dream of being a doctor had completely evaporated. It was a seriously hard moment and it felt like I'd never get over it.

Today, many years later, I'm grateful for that failure. Yes, really! Because what happened next is that I reapplied and studied hard to get the grades the second time. I developed resilience and other new skills along the way, meaning that when I got in the second time (smashed it!), I ended up doing really well all the way through medical school. Without the skills I'd developed by having to retake my exams, I might not have done so well.

So, while it's important to prepare as best we can for exams, remember that **everyone fails sometimes – and sometimes, in the long run, it's for the best.**

School can feel crammed with spelling tests and maths quizzes, as well as the bigger exams. As we get older, assessments like driving tests, job interviews or big projects will continue to be a part of our lives. If we've been practising how to accept and handle them while at school, we are likely to approach them more calmly in the future.

As you get older, you'll also meet plenty of people who didn't necessarily do well at school exams – and realize that those people are often just as successful and happy as everyone else.

In fact, many successful people have failed plenty of times and got into the habit of accepting the failure, learning from it and moving on – it's all part of their success.

HABIT HACK: HABIT TRACKERS

Enough about exams! Let's think about *prizes* (and maybe a little about revision). Have you ever received a merit award? Maybe you won a trophy or got a badge for completing a difficult task. I don't know why, but there is something *so* nice about having something physical as a prize for hard work.

So why don't you start giving yourself prizes? If rewards are enjoyable and they motivate us and make us feel proud, why wait for someone else to give them to us? We should give ourselves awards every day!

This is why I recommend creating a **habit tracker.** This is a device (like a calendar or a notebook) that tracks all the times we complete a happy habit.

Say you want to read every day (good choice – I recommend books by . . . *ahem* . . . Dr Alex George!) then get a calendar and mark off each day when you have read.

Or maybe you want to revise each day for thirty minutes? You could colour in the little box on the calendar every day that you complete your revision time.

The aim is to create a chain of marks – like a row of X's or coloured boxes – and keep the chain going. When you do ten in a row, **reward yourself**. How you do this is up to you, but options include:

★ Playing the national anthem and having an award ceremony like you are at the Olympics.

★ Or put 'Ceeeelebrate good times, come on!' on the speakers in your house and make everyone dance. Then hand yourself a prize (how about a banana – two happy habits for the price of one) and say thank you very much to yourself, shake your own hand, high-five yourself and do a speech:

First of all, I would like to thank **ME**.
It wouldn't have been possible without **ME**, and I am so grateful for always having me there to help **ME** . . .

This gives you a little burst of achievement that will help you **STICK TO YOUR HABIT**.

HAPPY HABIT 8: MONEY SENSE

Money is a big part of the world we live in, but learning how to manage it can feel daunting or confusing. Don't worry — figuring out the basics is easier than you might think. And creating smart money habits now will help Future You a million times over.

Whether it's weekly pocket money or some lovely birthday cash folded into your card once a year, it doesn't matter how much money you have — it's about how you look after it. Deciding what to do with your own money is an act of independence . . . and knowing that you've made a sensible decision is a really good feeling.

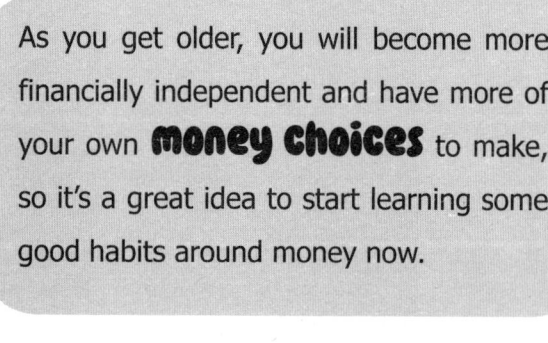

As you get older, you will become more financially independent and have more of your own **money choices** to make, so it's a great idea to start learning some good habits around money now.

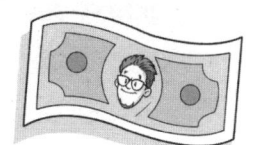

It can be tricky to make good choices at first, when money is a new and exciting thing to have, and there are so many things you can do with it. When I was ten, I used to get £1 a week pocket money, and I remember feeling annoyed when I tried to save up for my favourite car magazine but got tempted by sweets – so my money disappeared on those instead. A few moments of yumminess and then no magazine – rubbish!

As I grew older, I got better at saving. My first job was washing potatoes and dishes in a pub. It was quite dull, but I was so excited to earn my own money and save up for the moped I desperately wanted – and I did it!

MONEY TALKS

Let's start by thinking about some **common money terms** you might have heard. Good habits often need some good understanding to really work.

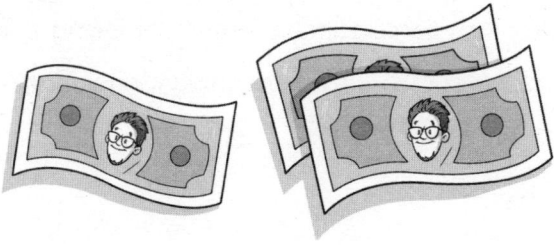

Cash is money that people can hold in their hand, so coins and banknotes. Cash is often kept in kept in piggy banks, or in a wallet or purse that people can take out and about with them. It's easy to keep track of how much cash someone has by just counting it.

A bank card is a card that people can use online or in person to pay for something, often by tapping on a card reader in a shop or restaurant. This can be a plastic card that someone holds or a card that's on their phone.

Bank cards are linked to **bank accounts**. It's important that everyone knows how much is in their bank account before they use a card, as if there isn't enough money, any payments may not be authorized, meaning that the person can't buy what they need.

People can check how much is in their bank account on an **app**, **online** or by **telephone banking**. Sometimes they may have to go to a **branch** too – this is the physical building of the bank.

Putting money in a bank account is called making a **deposit**. Taking the money out (including spending it on your card) is called making a **withdrawal**. Both of these are called

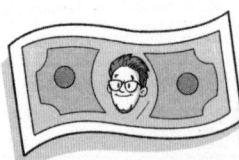

TRAnSACTiOnS, and they will show on a **bAnk STATemenT** – a list of all the activity on someone's account.

If you have a bank account, it will probably have money in it that a grown-up has deposited for you from their account – this could be your pocket money, birthday money, or money you've earned for chores around the house.

When you get a job, your employer will usually pay your **wAgeS** (the money you've earned for doing your job) directly into your bank account. Alternatively, they may pay you in cash.

BUDGETING

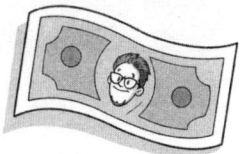

Have you heard of budgeting? This means keeping track of how much money you have – how much you've got coming in and how much you're spending.

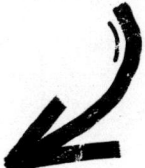

Budgeting encourages us to pause and think clearly about our money so that we can make the best choices around it. No matter how much money you or your family have right now, budgeting is an essential skill to help you stay in control of your money (rather than it controlling you!).

Here's a monthly budgeting exercise to try out.

Write the following column headings at the top of a sheet of paper:

Date	Amount	In or Out	Description	Total Amount

Every time you either receive or spend money, make a note of it. The **Total Amount** will go up and down each time.

Example:

Date	Amount	In or out	Description	Total Amount
1 May	£3	In	Pocket money	£3
5 May	£5	In	Money for chores	£8
6 May	£2	Out	Drink and snack	£6

At the end of the month, look over your entries and ask yourself some questions:

* Have you ended the month on a higher or lower total amount than the start of the month?

* How does it feel to see the amount of money going up or down?

* What in the 'out' column could you have saved? And how much would you have now if you hadn't spent it?

When you get older, you will be responsible for paying important bills, like gas and electricity for your home, food shopping, petrol, vet bills if you have a pet – all sorts of things. You will need to budget each month to check that you have enough money coming in from your job to pay all these bills. The more you've practised **budgeting** as a young person, the easier this will be as you get older – promise!

FUTURE YOU

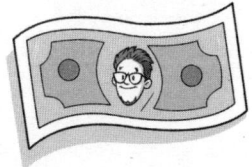

SAVING

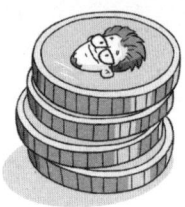

There's no getting around it – we live in a world where we're surrounded by tempting things to buy, from make-up to tech to fashion – and let's not forget the adverts constantly reminding us that these items are available. Experiences like going to the cinema or treating ourselves to a milkshake can also add up quickly, so it really helps to stay aware of when, how and *why* we are spending (especially if there isn't much spare money in our budget).

In my case, and you might not believe it – it's *protein bars*. I'm not kidding! When I decide I like a protein bar, I end up buying not one, not two, but **ten**. Whole boxes. Now this is partly a happy habit, because protein is *great* for our muscles, but well . . . ten boxes? I buy them because I like eating them, but I also have to be aware that I buy them because *I like the feeling of buying them.*

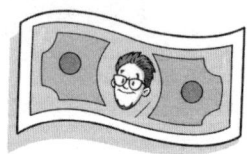

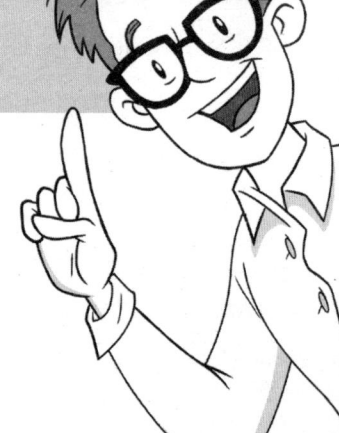

Sometimes buying things gives us a rush of dopamine (our old friend!), so we feel like we've earned a reward when really we should save our dopamine for happier, healthier habits.

You might also be facing peer pressure to buy the same things as your friends, even when each person in the group has a different amount of money available to them. We can't all have the same things, and we shouldn't, because we are individuals. **So try to appreciate what you *do* have rather than what you can't have.**

Also, try to remember that **the value you have as a person is not based on what you have or own.** Every person has equal value simply for being themselves. So whether someone has a new bike or an old one, shiny consoles or well-used board games, they are no better or worse than anybody else because of it.

So, if you have money to spend, hold on to it for things that you will truly enjoy or that will help you. If you spend your money just to fit in, you won't have any saved for the things that make you unique.

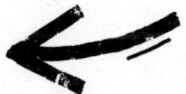

This might seem hard, but the best way to do it (and the happiest, most habitalicious way) is to start putting any money that's leftover after we've covered all our essential costs into *savings.* OK, so this might sound boring and pointless, but trust me, it's actually fun because we don't only get to save money for the things that we love, but we get to feel proud and confident in ourselves for doing it. It's just another way of making good choices *now* that lead to great things later.

SAVINGS EXERCISE

Choose an item that you **REALLY WANT** – the kind of thing you would ask for at Christmas. (Only this time, you're going to get it for yourself!)

Write down the price of it.

Make a plan of how you are going to get the money to buy it. There might be different ways of doing this, but remember that as part of the last exercise we looked at creating savings by *not* spending.

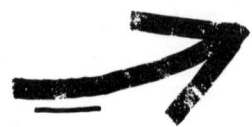

Here's an example:

That **T-shirt** that your mum refuses to buy for you cos 'you don't need any more clothes', but it's from your favourite brand, and you *reallllly* want it. **£10**

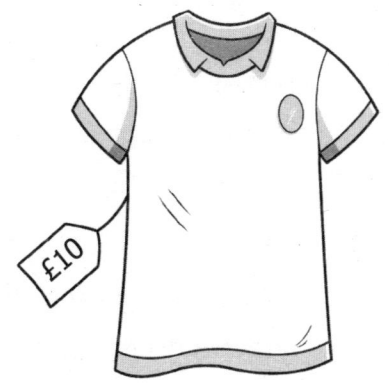

OPTION 1: Your pocket money is £2.50 a week. Save it for four weeks – which means not spending on anything else in that time. After four weeks, you can buy the T-shirt – result!

OPTION 2: Your pocket money is £2.50 a week. Save half of it for the T-shirt and spend half of it on other things. You can buy the T-shirt in eight weeks' time, which is fine by you as you'll enjoy some other treats in the meantime.

OPTION 3: Your pocket money is £2.50 a week. You want the T-shirt soon – ideally in time for your holiday in two weeks. So, as well as saving two weeks' pocket money (£5), you offer to do small jobs around the house for the next fortnight to quickly earn the remaining £5. Hoover the floors and wash the dirty dishes for two weeks, then it's shopping time!

However you choose to do it and however long it takes, saving up for something special is a really rewarding feeling. After all that waiting, it's great to get your hands on the item you worked so hard for.

Of course, there will be times when you slip up and don't save quite as much as you'd planned to, so it takes a little longer to save the full amount. There might also be times when money is tight at home and you don't get given any pocket money. That's fine – life and finances are unpredictable. But as long as we feel in control, and like we're doing our best around money most of the time, we're doing fine. The habit we want to avoid is spending without realizing we're doing it, then turning around one day and wondering where all our money went!

Saving 'for a rainy day' – in other words, for a time in the future where we might suddenly need some extra cash – is helpful too. This one can feel even harder because we don't actually know what it is we're saving for, but just putting aside even a pound per month for Future You is a kind and helpful thing to do for ourselves.

SAVINGS ACCOUNTS AND INTEREST

When you save money in a jar or piggy bank, you save exactly the amount you've put in.

Saving money in a bank account (or savings account) comes with an added perk – **interest**. This is an extra amount of money paid to you by the bank as a thank you for keeping your money with them. So every time you pay in some money to your account, you'll get a little top-up without having to do anything. I know what you're thinking: *Free money? Interrrresting.*

> The rate of interest differs from bank to bank, so you could ask an adult to help you find the best deal for you once you're ready to start saving.

But the coolest thing about interest is something called **compound interest.**

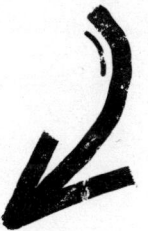

Every day we leave our savings in an account, we get paid a little bit more, and our savings grow. After they grow, the amount we get paid for those savings grows as well. On and on and on.

So let's say you put **£100** in a bank that gives you 10 per cent interest every year.

After 1 year: 10 per cent of £100 is £10, so now you have £110.

But after year 2: 10 per cent of £110 is £11, now you have £121.

Then after year 3: 10 per cent of £121 is £12.10, now you have £133.10.

This means that each year you're not *just* earning money on your first £100 – you're also earning money on the money *it* already earned. That's why it keeps growing faster!

You can think of it like an orchard with an apple tree, where each tree gives you apples with seeds that become trees of their own. Or maybe you like to think of it like our happy habits. Every day the progress we make grows more, because we use the progress from yesterday to go further today.

Famous physicist Albert Einstein once said,

> **Compound interest is the eighth wonder of the world.**

And who am I to argue with Einstein?

STAYING AWARE

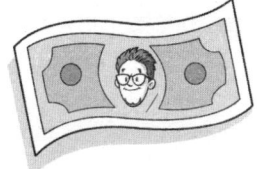

As you get older, it can be tempting to bury your head in the sand and avoid checking how much money you have in your bank account because it might cause you worry or stress if there's not enough in there. But trust me, ignoring your finances won't help anything – in fact, it can make things worse.

So stay aware of your money – how much you have, how much you want to save and how much you want to spend. These amounts will keep changing, but as long as you are keeping an eye on things, you'll be able to make the smartest decisions for you.

PART 5: JOY

HAPPY HABIT 9: GET CREATIVE

What do you enjoy watching or reading? Do you love superhero films or graphic novels? Do you prefer animation or stories about people from history?

How does watching or reading the things you love make you feel?

I ask this because creating feelings in other people is one of the best things about creativity. We humans invent and imagine things, and then give enjoyment and inspiration to other people who come across them.

That's pretty incredible. Look, I love the other creatures we share our planet with, but you've got to admit that creativity is something that makes *humans* special. I have not seen a dog do a sculpture, and I am not a fan of any songs recorded by rabbits.

Have you ever created something? How did it make you feel?

Maybe you don't really think of writing a story or doing a painting as creative, but if there was nothing on a page before you arrived and something when you finished, then well done, you've created something!

Maybe you don't feel strongly about the word 'creativity'? Or you aren't sure that you are a creative person?

I used to think that being creative only meant you were brilliant at art. That you probably had your own easel and a load of paints and spent your spare time in a field painting sunflowers while wearing a paint-splattered outfit.

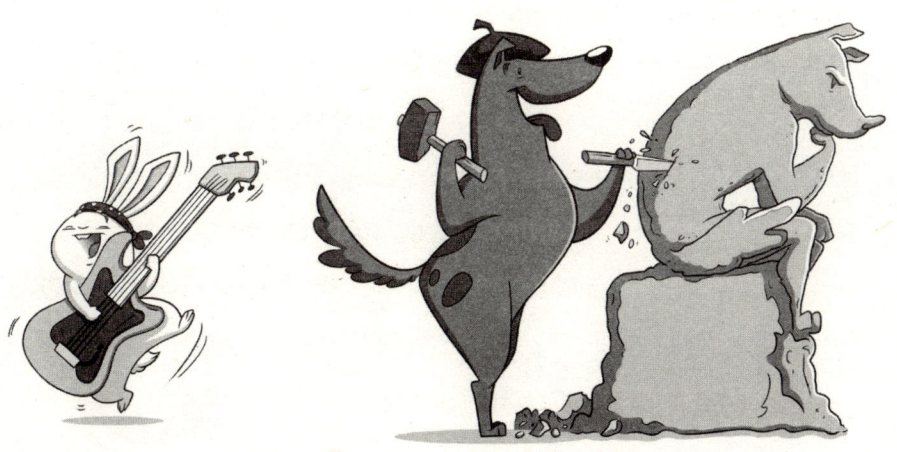

In other words, not me. Then, as time went by, I realized that there were so many ways to be creative. Here are a few that I didn't know were creative until later. Give yourself a little high five if you have ever done one!

- ♥ Making up a **song** (even if it is meant to be silly)
- ♥ Inventing a **game** with your friends
- ♥ Playing a **character** (any funny voice will do)
- ♥ Doing an **impression**
- ♥ **Dancing**
- ♥ Doing **tricks** with a ball
- ♥ Making a **joke**
- ♥ Playing a **prank**
- ♥ Imagining a **character** (this could be a monster, an alien, a new animal or your teacher – as a monster, alien or new animal!)

My point is that we tend to think creativity is about skills or jobs, like painter or singer, writer or guitarist. So creativity ends up sounding like *work.*

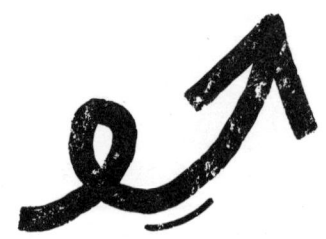

When in reality, creativity is *mostly* about fun, and most things that are fun involve creativity. Solutions to difficult problems require us to get creative, as do making plans for the weekend and imagining our future self too.

So, our first step is to realize *all* the ways in which we are creative. Like me, you might not be a great artist, but you are *definitely creative.* So take a moment to go through the list I have given opposite and think of all the ways your creativity shines, and feel free to add a few of your own. Maybe even make up some imaginary things you *could do* (which is creativity in action!).

Because everyone has creativity, it's part of being human. And from a mental health point of view, it's very good for us to tap into that part of our nature. Creativity helps connect the two hemispheres of your brain – the left 'logical' side and the right 'emotional' side – and keeps your brain functioning well as a whole. So don't listen to people who say you're either a left-brained person OR a right-brained person. You have a whole brain, *thank you very much.*

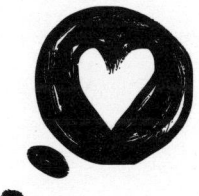

OK, SOUNDS GREAT. BUT WHAT WILL WORK FOR ME?

Well, the great thing is that you get to decide. You get to find your preferred forms of creativity based on what you enjoy doing. So think about the ways in which you either play with your friends or entertain yourself alone.

Do you like inventing games or characters? Maybe creative writing or drama will be something you enjoy.

Do you like making things or seeing how different parts fit together? Maybe you should start with Lego and think about building more complex things.

Whether you enjoy a good song, book, dance or joke, there are no rules, and no right or wrong ways to be creative. Just have fun, without anyone telling you how to, and you are being creative.

So **get creative about being creative**. It doesn't have to be something offered to you at a school club – you can figure out your own thing. For example, I love science, but I also love creating video content. One day, I realized I could combine the two, so I started exploring creative ways to teach medical science. I made some videos with a GoPro camera about how to examine and assess knee injuries. Awesome!

As well as my 'science-y' creativity, I write books, draw on my iPad and play the guitar – as well as listening to both rock and classical music to unwind.

MAKE CREATIVITY A HAPPY HABIT

Below are a few pointers for building your creative habits in a stress-free way. But before we get started, remember this: while it's healthy to take pleasure in improving at something, we shouldn't ever feel under pressure to be 'the best'.

We can learn the piano because it makes our heart sing, and it's fun to bash out Christmas tunes for our friends to sing along to. We can mess around with pipe cleaners or doodle with felt tips for hours without expecting our creations to be displayed in an art gallery. We can make up silly stories that make us happy without anyone else in the world ever laying eyes on them.

Besides, art is what we would call **subjective** – meaning that one famous painting loved by millions might leave some people thinking, *what's the big deal?* The same goes for popular songs and books. You and your friends probably have different tastes in all sorts of things. So what you create might be someone else's cup of tea or not, but that's not important.

CHOOSE YOUR HABIT

It could be something you do already, that you'd like to do more of, or something you're trying out for the first time. Let's say it's creative writing. Perhaps you keep a diary, or maybe you've enjoyed writing a short story in English and dream of writing a book one day but have no idea how to start.

As with all of these habits, the best way to do this is – you guessed it! – to . . . **start**. Find yourself a comfy place to sit. Surround yourself with some cushions, your favourite books to inspire you and some snacks. Whatever feels good for you – every writer has their own way of doing things!

Find a good time, when you're not distracted by anything and not in a rush. Then, just make a start.

Remember, your brain might need a little help at first.

Here's where you can help your brain out. Prove to it that you are a writer, by writing some words down. It doesn't matter what they are. Just aim for five sentences.

Even if you're just writing something like,

'Hello, blank notebook. My name is Alex George, and I don't know what to write. Help? Help. **Helppppppp**.'

Five sentences, **done**. You've started your habit!

You've shown your brain that you can write, and it will stimulate the release of dopamine, encouraging you to do it again. And it will feel slightly more possible next time you do it. New ideas will be more likely to flow because you've overcome the first hurdle of doing it, and your brain will be less preoccupied with feeling scared that you can't.

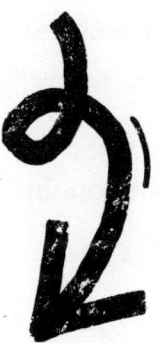

The same applies to writing music — just think of a line of a song and you're on the way. Or creating art by doodling a shape on a page.

KEEP IT LIGHT AND FUN

The trick to keep this habit going is not to worry about what you're writing (or creating). It's unlikely that you'll casually jot down a whole book on your first try. You might end up with loads of random bits and bobs, and some half-developed ideas. Some might be destined for the bin, never to be looked at again, but some might be the spark of something that ends up taking a life of its own.

THE GOOD, THE BAD AND THE COMPLETELY RANDOM – IT'S ALL PART OF THE PROCESS.

It's something I've been thinking a lot about since I interviewed bestselling children's author Jacqueline Wilson on my *Stompcast* podcast a couple of years ago. Jacqueline spoke about how she'd loved making up stories from a young age. Aged nine, a teacher gave all the kids a new school notebook to fill however they pleased. Jacqueline wrote about twenty pages of a novel – an amazing first start at that age.

Decades later, she has written hundreds of successful books.

Jacqueline also mentioned a great writing tip: 'I always tell children that you can use other people's characters. They can write a story about Tracy Beaker if they want.' It's something Jacqueline has done herself, making up extra bits about characters from *The Magic Faraway Tree* books by Enid Blyton and the family in *The Railway Children* by E. Nesbit in her book *The Primrose Railway Children*.

It's great advice, especially on days when you're feeling totally stuck. I like to imagine new adventures for one of my favourite characters – Harry Potter. There are so many things he could get up to on any given day!

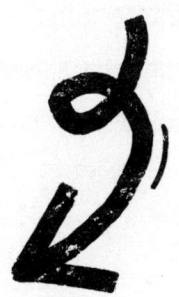

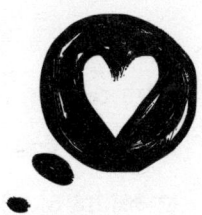

So, if you're feeling completely stuck for ideas, why not use a favourite book as a springboard, then write a brand-new chapter for fun? How about a different ending from the original one? It will give you a structure to work with and give your imagination a good workout at the same time.

This can apply to other creative habits too. Draw a new adventure for your favourite comic-book character, put a new twist on a banana bread recipe, or write a new verse for your favourite song. There is always something out there for you to be inspired by.

You could even team up with a friend. If the habit is writing, you could write a chapter, pass it to them to write the next one – then back to you. This might feel less daunting, and more fun, than doing it alone. Imagine what you could cook up between you!

THE FINISHED PRODUCT

After putting your creative habit into action for a few weeks or months, you may have something to show for it. A few chapters of a first draft? A book full of sketches? A brand-new jumper that you've knitted from scratch?

This can feel so satisfying – and it should. It's tangible evidence of the hard work and commitment you've made to your new habit. It might even be something beautiful that you're proud to display to others. BUT . . .

You also might not end up with something like this. Don't worry if that's the case. It's not about perfect results, or any results, really – besides the massive win of relaxation and stress-reduction!

Unless you *really* haven't enjoyed the process . . .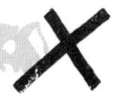

If your habit continues to feel like an uphill struggle, it may be a sign to try a different one. The only way to know for sure if something is right for you is to spend some time on it. It doesn't mean you have to commit to it for life. Maybe you try calligraphy but then find out you're naturally having more fun with your sibling's Lego – and decide to build a whole city. Great!

As well as being a happy habit that will benefit you in the moment, working on your creativity will help you out in the future. It will teach you how to look at a problem from different angles and come up with **creative solutions** – whether you are stuck on something in your job, or in your personal life.

For example, once I had to give a talk at a school, but I really wanted my message to reach more kids. I'd put a lot of work into preparing the talk, and I knew that lots of kids would find it helpful, but obviously I could only be in one place at a time! So, I came up with the idea of livestreaming my talk to 20,000 kids around the country.

My *Stompcast* podcast came about because I knew I wanted to interview guests, but there were lots of podcasts doing that already. So I came up with a creative spin on the interview format: as well as interviewing a guest, I would combine it with my hobby of walking in nature. It took a bit of brainpower to figure out how the recordings would work outdoors, but ultimately the idea worked really well.

Nurturing our creativity is something that gets even harder to make time for as we get older and busier with other commitments. But if we've got into the habit as a young person, we will tap in more naturally to our **creative brain** in spite of whatever else is going on – and reap the benefits for life!

HAPPY HABIT 10: THE JOY OF GIVING BACK AND HELPING OTHERS

This is one of the happiest habits imaginable. When we do kind things for others, we make them happy, which makes us happy, which only makes us want to go and do it again. It's like **kindness is a form of renewable energy** that gains power and momentum when we give it a try.

You can start by practising this with people you know and love, but the goal is to create the habit of helping the wider community. This is how we make a start on **improving the whole world**.

It's amazing how much change one person (you!) can make in the world, helping improve people's lives in all sorts of brilliant ways. I'm not talking about anything grand here – you don't have to change your whole life. I'm talking about small acts of kindness that we can work into our daily routine, and that will cause a ripple effect of positivity.

Because if you do something kind for someone, they're more likely to do something kind for someone else. You can inspire others with your actions, which in itself is a powerful thing.

IT FEELS GOOD TO DO GOOD

Have you ever done something nice for someone and felt a warm feeling wash over you? Maybe you let someone have the last brownie because they were having a bad day, even though it was extra-gooey and delicious, and you *reallllllly* wanted it. Or maybe you chose someone to join your sports team to cheer them up, even though they weren't necessarily the best player left, then lit up when you saw their reaction.

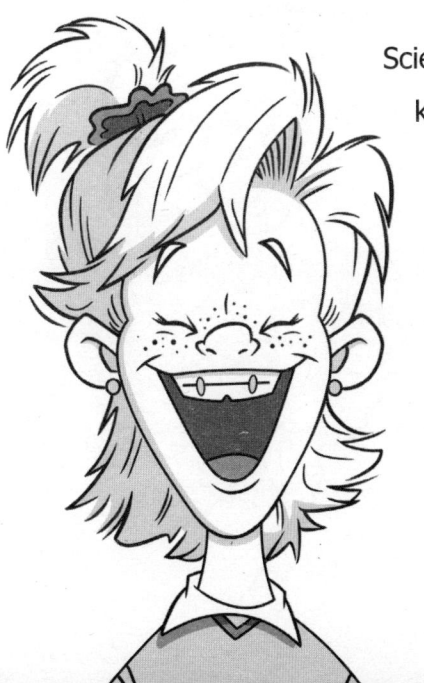

Science shows us this is because acts of kindness release feel-good hormones including **dopamine** and **serotonin** (thanks, brain). As humans, we're designed to look after our tribe, as we're more likely to survive and flourish as a team. So we're hardwired to help each other, and it feels brilliant to be kind.

It's one of the reasons I love being a doctor. I get to experience helping people every day – it feels rewarding simply because I'm making a difference to people's lives. Sometimes my shift in the A&E unit would put things into perspective for me when I had problems or stresses at home. I'd see that everyone has bad days – which is probably why they ended up meeting me in the A&E department! – and I'd realize that we all have bad luck sometimes. But because we're human, we have the amazing power to help each other work through the tough times.

WHERE DO I START?

With the best will in the world, it can be hard to know how to get started with acts of kindness. So here's an easy one to kick us off: **smiling!**

You might not always feel in the mood to do this, of course, but if you are having a good day, why not share that energy with someone walking past? Think of it the other way around – have you ever been in a grumpy mood then found yourself randomly smiling when you see someone else smiling or laughing? This happens because smiles are contagious – and proven to lift our mood – so spreading them around is something we can all do from time to time.

The same goes for **thanking people**. It makes them feel seen, which is always a good feeling. So, if someone holds the door for you or picks up the pen you dropped and hands it back, say thank you to let them know it's appreciated. That little moment of connection will improve their day and yours.

You can even give out more random 'thank you's – thank you for being you. Thanks for being here today. Everyone loves a thank you!

Maybe you want to go further and decide to start putting kind words out into the world whenever you can. Friendly compliments like, 'I like your shoes,' or 'You're doing a great job,' can really make someone feel noticed. You never know when someone is having a hard day, and your words might have been the best thing in it.

Observing people and situations around us is key to this chapter. **The more we practise looking around at things, the better our brains get at noticing if there is anyone who might need a hand.**

Say your PE teacher is busy gathering up tennis balls at the end of your lesson. Instead of running off with your friends without a second thought, why not grab a few to help? Your teacher is likely to be grateful, and you can catch up with your friends a minute or two later.

After lunch in the canteen, you could clear a few plates or throw some used napkins in the bin on your way out.

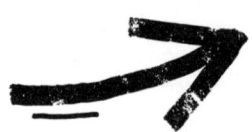

If you spot a new pupil looking lost in the hallway, offer to help them find their way to their next class. It's hard to ask for help sometimes, particularly when you're the new kid! So be the person who steps in nice and early to offer help. In many of these cases the skill we are practising is **empathy**. This is the ability to imagine what it must feel like to be the other person. If you have ever been the new kid at a school or in a group, you will be able to imagine what other people are going through and be understanding.

Best of all, when you learn the skill of empathy, even the hard moments in your life can start to feel useful. Try it next time you are feeling down in the dumps. Say you feel left out – instead of only thinking about how hard it is for you, focus on how this will help you to understand other people who are left out in the future. Or if someone ever helps you in a difficult moment, remember to learn to hold on to how that made you feel and use it as a reminder to do the same for other people who might need help.

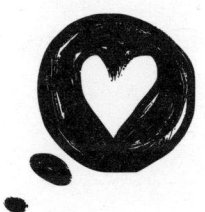

The more you notice these little opportunities, the more you will find yourself doing things like this automatically. Kindness will become a happy habit, people will be kinder to you, and you will learn how to help yourself and others when times are tough.

Remember, your amazing brain is adapting all the time, so you can be a great teacher *to yourself.*

YOUR WIDER COMMUNITY

While you probably spend a lot of your time at school — making it a *great* place to work on this habit daily — there are plenty of opportunities outside school to make positive changes.

And when it comes to after school, weekends and holidays, we can put more time and planning into potential acts of kindness too.

Here are some ideas to get you started, but you are definitely the best person to dream up things that will work for you!

⭐ Offer to walk your neighbour's dog.

⭐ Cook something yummy for an elderly neighbour.

⭐ Hold a bake sale to raise money for a charity of your choice.

⭐ Sort out some of your old clothes/toys/books and take them to the charity shop so someone else can enjoy them AND you can raise money for a good cause. Double bubble!

⭐ Collect some canned goods from your neighbours for the local food bank. (You could offer to do small jobs in return.)

⭐ Write to your school's youth council – or even your local MP! – to raise awareness about a cause you feel strongly about. This is a way of letting people in positions of power know what you think they should be doing.

⭐ Do a sponsored silence or draw-a-thon (where you draw non-stop for a couple of hours, so get your pens ready!) to raise money for charity.

Write to someone you admire, like your favourite author or illustrator, to let them know how much you enjoy their work – it will make their day!

You could schedule one '**giving back**' activity in every school holiday. It's a great habit to get into, and one that will grow naturally the more you do it.

Over time, people will start to view you as not just kind but trustworthy and someone who can be relied on. This can help you build strong relationships with those around you – a life skill Future You will be extremely grateful for.

HABIT HACK: TEMPTATION BUNDLING

Another habit hack for you, and this is a good one. If you have a habit you struggle to stick to, bundle it up with something you find easy.

Maybe you want to find extra motivation to do some of the good deeds mentioned above. Well, take the example of the

draw-a-thon – if you enjoy drawing, then this is an example of bundling, as you will be doing something that you enjoy that *also* helps you keep up the habit of being kind.

Say you struggle to remember to clean your room, but you love listening to your **favourite tunes**. Then clean while you listen to your favourite music.

Maybe you *want* to exercise but you'd rather watch **cartoons**. So watch cartoons while doing star jumps!

This means that your natural habits – the things you do without thinking – encourage you to do the ones that you might forget!

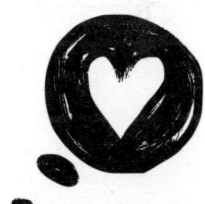

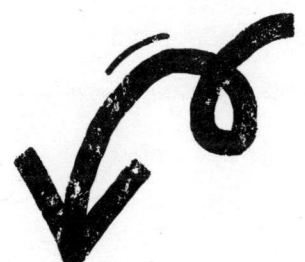

PART 6: CONNECT

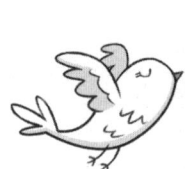

HAPPY HABIT 11: CONNECTING WITH NATURE

Aaaahhhh, the great outdoors. Wind in your hair, mud on your boots, your dog on a lead (this is important if you are in the woods, to protect nesting birds).

As I've mentioned before, there is nothing I love more than moving around in nature. It makes me feel calm but also raises my energy levels. It makes me feel happy, but also offers time to think. I may be surrounded by trees, but it is the place where I feel most free.

You see, most of us live in a pretty controlled modern world. Cross the road when the green man appears. Wake up when your alarm tells you to. Sit down and do as you are told. A lot of this is for our own good, but it sometimes leaves us craving **a time and space where we are *free.***

A space where there aren't signs and rules, and where  we can do as we please, as long as we are respectful.

That place is out there in the natural world. In a local green space or fields, by the sea or on a hilltop we can feel free, grow healthier and find calm. I spend a lot of my time trying to explain the benefits of getting into the natural world, because as a doctor and mental-health ambassador I know how good it is for us, but as a person, *I feel it.*

So let's look at why nature is so important to our minds and bodies.

Many thousands of years ago, we were all extremely connected to nature. Early humans relied on nature for food (by hunting and gathering) and to make clothes, shelters and tools. For them, nature was survival and, because of this, they probably felt deeply connected to it every second of the day. They *were* nature, just as much as the animals they hunted and the rocks they made their tools from.

As time went on and human societies made incredible advances, this deep connection to the outdoors was slowly disrupted when people started to build homes and settle in one place, when towns and cities sprang up and, most recently, when new technology came along.

Nowadays, as we connect to our screens and devices in our cosy homes, it can feel like a bit of an effort to break away from all that entertainment and get outside, relax and just . . . breathe. Something that happened naturally for our ancestors has become something we often forget to do, or don't really want to do, because it's so easy and convenient for us to stay indoors. But remember, we don't have to go far to feel the benefits of being outdoors – just a trip to a local park with your parent or caregiver is enough to help you connect with the natural world.

But deep down, our human need to be in nature hasn't changed. The reality that we are *animals* from the natural world has not changed. It's how we were always meant to be, which is why you will often feel your mood lifting soon after leaving the house.

WHY NATURE IS GOOD FOR OUR BRAINS

Studies show that spending regular time in green spaces is a surefire way to reduce stress, anxiety (worry) and feeling sad.

It also boosts our **cognitive function** (how well our brain works) and helps us to sleep better at night. In nature, we're more likely to feel positive emotions like calmness and contentment, and we find it easier to concentrate.

As a child playing in the fields of Wales, I always felt grounded in nature and **I make an effort now to turn to nature whenever life feels tricky**. Connecting to nature at a young age builds the habit for when you're older, which is why I'm encouraging you to get out there as much as possible now. The natural world is waiting for you!

Even if you don't live in the countryside, you can usually find access to green spaces, from a garden or park to a nature reserve or woods in your local area. Many local councils plant street trees and roadside wildflowers – are there any near where you live?

NATURE HABIT 1: LIGHT UP YOUR MORNINGS

The internal 24-hour clock that runs your body is called your **circadian rhythm,** and all living things, including plants and animals, have one. It tells you when to wake up and when to go to sleep, as well as affecting your mood and how you digest your food.

Your circadian rhythm responds to light and darkness, and it can get messed up if, for example, you stay up really late or travel to a different time zone – this is how jetlag comes about. Changes to your circadian rhythm leave you feeling groggy during the day and wide awake at bedtime.

One of the most helpful things we can do to support our body clock is to expose ourselves to natural light when we wake up. This will signal to our brains that it's morning. Of course, back when we were all living in caves, this would have happened naturally as it shone into the cave opening! Here are a couple of easy ways to help your body wake up naturally:

 As soon as you wake up, get out of bed and open your curtains or blinds. Whatever you do next – even if it's getting back into bed for a few minutes – relax and feel the daylight on your face and skin.

 After breakfast, spend a few minutes in your garden, balcony or any space outside your home, or go for a ten-minute walk (this could be a walk to school).

With these easy steps, you will feel your mind and body gently start to wake up, like a flower unfurling. The longer you can absorb natural light and avoid artificial light from screens in the morning, the better.

NATURE HABIT 2: CONNECT WITH NATURE THROUGHOUT THE DAY

As the day progresses, look for other chances to connect with nature. These will depend on where you live, and what your normal routine is. Let's be honest, a full day's rambling through the countryside won't be possible most of the time. The trick is to look around and enjoy glimmers of nature throughout our day, bringing us small moments of calm and boosting our well-being each time.

It's amazing what you can spot once you start looking.

THROUGH THE SEASONS

IN SPRING

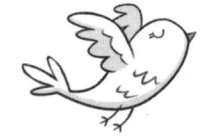

🌿 Seek out the new pink or white **blossom** appearing on the trees. Sniff it to see if it's fragrant.

🌿 Go on a **bee-spotting** walk – head for areas with plenty of flowers!

🌿 Plant some **sunflower seeds** (late April will give them enough time to grow by summer).

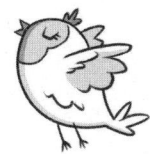

IN SUMMER

(remembering that SPF we talked about earlier):

🌱 Kick off your shoes and feel the **grass** under your feet.

🌱 Read a book or have a **lovely snooze** under the shade of a big, leafy tree.

🌱 If you visit a **beach**, enjoy the feeling of the sand and the cold splash of seawater on your toes. Collect some interesting shells and pebbles, and notice how they've been smoothed down by the water.

IN AUTUMN

🌱 Go for a **stroll** and challenge yourself to find five different colours in nature.

🌱 Crunch through a pile of fallen **leaves**, listening to the rustle they make.

IN WINTER

🌿 Bundle up in some warm clothes and head **OUTSIDE**, noticing how invigorating the fresh, cold air is to breathe. Bonus points if you can see your own breath!

🌿 Notice the shape of the **frost** patterns on the ground, on trees and parked cars.

ALL YEAR ROUND

🌿 Look up and watch the **clouds** for a few minutes. Can you spot any interesting shapes or notice the clouds moving across the sky?

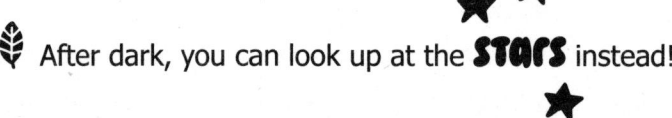

🌿 After dark, you can look up at the **stars** instead!

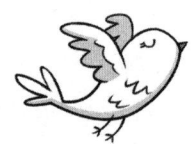

INDOORS

If going out isn't always an option, there are plenty of ways to connect with nature in your home.

♥ Looking after **houseplants** became a source of comfort to many people during the Covid lockdowns, and it's no surprise. Some scientists think that caring for plants could trigger a release of **oxytocin**, the hormone that makes us feel relaxed, while simply being around greenery has the same benefits as it does outdoors. There's nothing like a new baby leaf sprouting from the plant you've been carefully watering and monitoring for weeks.

♥ Always look after a houseplant according to the instructions. Make sure it has enough water, the right kind of soil and is in an area where it receives enough light, then take pride in watching it thrive. You could even decorate its pot with stickers and give your plant pet a name! (Barry the fern? Ange the chilli plant? Lily the . . . lily?)

♥ Watch **nature documentaries**, like *Blue Planet* and *Planet Earth* with David Attenborough – plus many others. These are great for sparking curiosity, as you'll find out about nature far from home and discover all sorts of weird and wonderful animal species living under water and above land. Visually, these documentaries are a treat for the eyes, which helps!

♥ Listen to **nature sounds** on an app. This will help you enjoy the calming power of birdsong or rushing waterfalls, from home.

The brilliant thing about nature is that the more you look around, the more you'll become aware of – there is just so much to explore.

NATURE HABIT 3: NATURE JOURNALLING

Writing down or drawing some of the things you've seen or experienced in nature is a wonderful way to keep enjoying them.

🌿 In a **notebook or journal**, list five ways you've connected with nature at the end of every week.

🌿 Take a notebook out with you when you're heading to an outdoor space, and sketch some trees, flowers, clouds or insects – anything that **inspires** you. Add the date, and you'll have a beautiful reminder of what you saw that day.

🌿 Do a **leaf rubbing** (this is a really good one to do in autumn). Collect a few leaves with different shapes (spiky or rounded, for example) and take them home. Cover each one with a sheet of paper and rub over the paper with a crayon, to transfer the leaf's pattern on to the paper.

After a few months of nature journalling, you can look back and see if you can spot the seasons changing through your entries. It's incredibly grounding to **pay attention to the natural world changing around us,** as it is so much bigger than us and puts our own problems into perspective.

Whatever uncertainties we might be facing, the leaves will always change colour in autumn, and blossom will always appear in spring – fact!

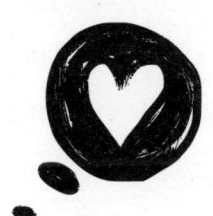

HAPPY HABIT 12: FRIENDSHIP FUN

Do you know who else is a part of nature that we can connect to? Other people. I don't mean that your friend from football is *actually* a tree, or that most of your class are wild animals (although . . . sometimes). I just mean that **friendship is in our nature**. We were born to connect with other people – it's free, it's a laugh and it's good for us.

WHAT MORE CAN WE ASK FOR FROM OUR HAPPY HABITS?

Having fun with our friends is key to a happy life. They know us in a special way, make us smile, provide a safe space for us to share our problems, and encourage us to try new things – maybe rollerblading, a new game or a pizza topping we haven't tried before. Through the highs and lows, I have learned so much from my friends over the years. And I've also learned that nurturing those friendships is a habit worth its weight in gold.

WHAT'S YOUR FRIENDSHIP STYLE?

Friendships look different for everyone. Some people are more **introverted** – meaning they feel most comfortable socializing with one or two trusted friends, as well as enjoying time alone. Others are more **extroverted** – those who feel energized by large groups of people and prefer to spend most of their time with others. The chances are you may be a bit of both, depending on what kind of a day you're having!

Whatever your friendship circle looks like, close social connection is something most of us can't do without. As human beings, we evolved as part of a tribe, sticking together for safety and survival – and that's why it feels good to be in the presence of our friends. Just being around each other is usually relaxing, even if we're not doing anything particularly special.

Developing solid friendships is a lifelong habit that will serve us well in the future as we meet new people in different life settings – and continue to enjoy the friendships we already have. Many adults stay in touch with people they met at school and count them among their most treasured friends. I also love the idea that there are friends out there that I haven't met yet – what they are up to right now, and when will we cross paths for the first time?

In this chapter, we'll learn about healthy friendship habits: how to show up for our friends, plan fun stuff together, check in on them if they're going through a hard time, celebrate their wins and shower them in gratitude for being so amazing!

WHY FRIENDS ARE GOOD FOR US

It's been scientifically proven that hanging out with our mates is actually good for our health. It's just as important as healthy nutrition and staying active, and increases our chances of living longer.

Being around people we like and trust lowers our stress levels and can even have a positive impact on our immune system. When you're lonely for long periods of time, your white blood cells change their behaviour, leading to more inflammation in your body.

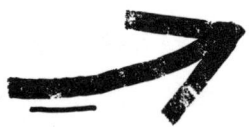

Oxytocin is one of the key bonding hormones. It's produced by our brains and released into our bloodstreams when we see, hear, smell or cuddle our loved ones. It's important for the bonding between a newborn baby and its parents, and it is also linked to our friendships and romantic relationships.

When oxytocin is released by chatting or sharing a hug with a friend, we feel trusting and relaxed. Scientists think you can feel the benefits of this happy hormone just by talking or thinking about a close pal.

Having lots of small, positive interactions with one or several friends on a daily basis makes us feel connected and loved. Of course, there's no such thing as a perfect friendship, and you might sometimes have fall-outs with your mates – that's totally normal.

The key is to always keep looking for **fun and meaningful connection** wherever we can.

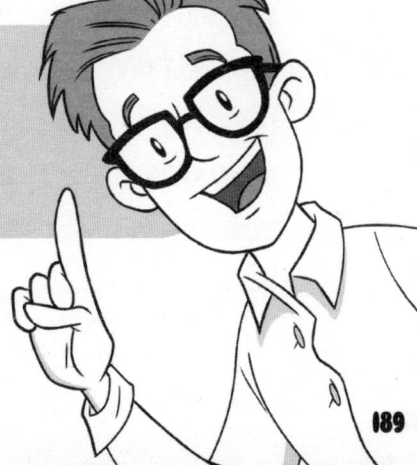

CHOOSING FRIENDS AND BEING INCLUSIVE

Sometimes we might want to befriend the popular kid in class, or the one who has the coolest clothes and the best parties.

In my experience, this isn't the best way to choose our friends. They should be people who will stick with you in difficult times and celebrate your wins, no matter what kind of trainers either of you have. So look for people who take an interest in you and your hobbies and are genuinely keen to get to know you. And if they throw great parties, then . . . hey, that's a bonus.

It may take a little while to figure out who this person is for you and that's OK – in the meantime, try chatting to lots of people. Don't assume you won't get on with someone or have anything in common, as it's impossible to know for sure until you get to know them. You may find out that you both have a shared interest, or just a similar way of thinking about the world.

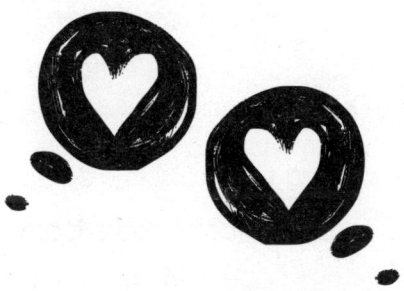

Our friends don't have to be the same as us, but we want them to be a good match. This means helping us enjoy the good times and feel stronger in the hard ones.

I didn't really find a group in primary school. I hated being tall because I stood out from everyone else. I could also feel like an outsider because I was naturally quite shy and sensitive. Later, I realized it was a good thing to be unique. My sensitive side, as it turned out, made me a good doctor and communicator.

In the meantime, I got to know lots of people and in Year 9, I met my best friend, Adam, who is still my best friend today. We had the same sense of humour, and he's been there for me in the good times and the bad. We feel comfortable having honest conversations and telling each other to wise up if we need to!

When we were both in Year 10, I decided I wanted to be a doctor, and he decided to become a dentist. So far, so good. Then one day, we had to have our BCG injections (vaccinations against a disease called tuberculosis). Guess what happened? We *both* fainted. It turned out he was a future dentist who was scared of needles, and I was a doctor in waiting who had the same problem!

Remember we spoke about **empathy** when we discussed the power of kindness? Well, it's super important in good friendships and in making new ones. When we are empathetic, we understand how our friends are feeling, and that means we can support them better than ever. Sometimes, my friends know what I need even better than I do.

Empathy is also a skill that helps us see when people might *need* a friend.
It could be someone new to the school, or someone who faces certain challenges, or just hasn't made any friends yet.

What would you like someone else to do if you were in the outsider's situation? Maybe just say hello. Or invite them to sit with you at lunch or ask if they want to join in the rounders game after school. You don't know how they will react, so don't worry if they say, 'No, thanks.' More often than not, you might well have turned someone's day around with a friendly remark, and one day you might be grateful if someone does the same for you.

The more you do these little actions to welcome people in, the more of a habit it will become, and you'll get used to that nice buzz of having done something kind for someone. You'll probably make some new friends in the process too!

SPENDING QUALITY TIME TOGETHER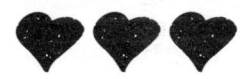

It's likely that we see a lot of our friends at school – and enjoy hanging out after school or on weekends too. But sometimes we can get bogged down with homework, activities or family stuff and struggle to carve out proper space for our friends.

So, the habit to build here is making quality time for our friends on a regular basis. This is good for our own well-being as well as theirs. Having a right old giggle with our friends reminds us not to take life too seriously – and while messaging each other is fun, hanging out in person is even better for us. It's how we create memories that we will go on to cherish for years to come.

This does take some planning, and I'd encourage you to **be the person that reaches out** and does the inviting. It may feel like a lot of effort, and sometimes we all worry that people will say no, but if you're real friends, you'll always be able to make some sort of plan to get together.

I've had times when I'm really busy at work and haven't seen one of my friends in weeks, or even months. I catch myself thinking, *I miss them – why haven't they made an effort?* Then realize it's up to me to reply to their message! It happens to us all, but as long as we can get into the habit of making the effort at least some of the time, our friendships will survive the busy periods.

Here are a few ideas for weekend or school-holiday fun you could suggest:

♥ a **picnic** in the park

♥ a **movie** or **board-games** night

♥ a **kickabout** followed by a **gaming session**

♥ an **adventure day** when you try something new together or go to a new place

♥ a **'yes day'**, when you have to do everything your friend suggests – and then next time it's your turn!

LISTEN UP

The more time we spend with our friends, the more likely we are to open up to each other about any worries or concerns we have in our lives. Learning to trust someone with our 'stuff' is an important part of friendship. That stuff may be to do with bullying, body image, stress, exams, family issues or something else.

So remember to listen up if your friend is telling you something important – give them your full attention. You don't have to have the answer to their problems – in fact, we rarely do (even grown-ups!).

Just being a kind and supportive listening ear when they are getting something off their chest is a big help.

It's nice to keep checking in with a friend who has shared a problem too, to remind them that you are a safe space for them. Or if they haven't opened up but you think there might be something on their mind, you could ask them if they'd like to chat about anything. Hopefully, they will do the same for you when you are going through something tricky. That's exactly what friends are for – **life throws all kinds of things at us, good and bad – and it's wonderful to have someone by our side for all of it.**

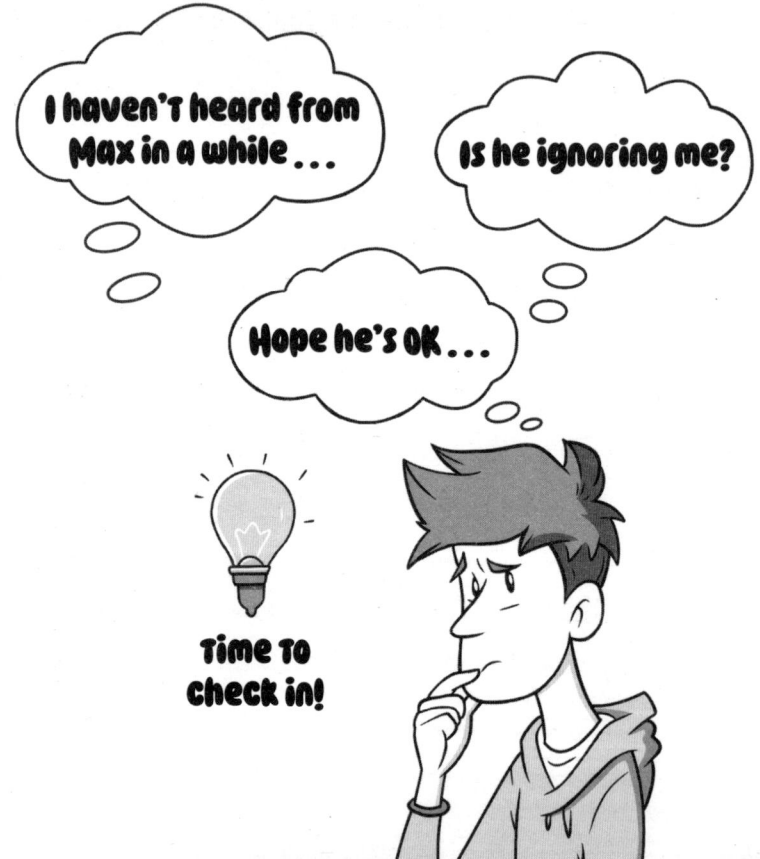

CELEBRATING OUR FRIENDS

As well as making sure we spend plenty of time together, we can celebrate our friends in other ways too:

♥ Write a list showing all of your friends' birthdays. Check it regularly to see whose is coming up, and then make a special card or gift for them.

♥ If you have a friend who lives far away, send them a postcard full of the latest gossip or plan a meet-up in the holidays.

♥ If a friend is ill or going through a tough time, you could put together a little 'thinking of you' bundle – this could include their favourite snack, a friendship bracelet and a handwritten note with funny doodles to cheer them up.

♥ Similarly, if they have done something brilliant, you could make them a gift showing how proud of them you are – or even throw them a surprise party!

Have a think about the person, or people, in your life who are most deserving of some special attention, then take it from there. Whether they are friends or family (family can be friends too!), you will both feel glad that you have made a special effort for them.

HABIT HACK: COMMITMENT REMINDERS

We feel happy by connecting with nature and other people but we also feel happier and more able to stick to our habits if we connect the easy ones and the hard ones together.

We spoke earlier about **habit bundling** – how we can do two things side by side (music and cleaning, cartoons and exercises). But we can also make our fun things *depend* on healthy, harder ones too.

For example (and I know this may seem hard for you gamers) – give your video-game controller to your parents or carers and say, 'Only give this back after I finish my homework.'

Perhaps you want to learn a new skill, like drawing. Put your pencil case out as a reminder to have a go after school. Then, every time you pass it, you'll remember to practise.

Or create **social reminders**.

Other people can help you stick to your good habits by cheering you on or watching you. Why does this work? Because we all care what others think – we like making people proud, and we don't want to let them down.

Here's how social reminders work:

1. You tell a friend or family member what habit you're working on.

2. They check in on you, or you check in with them.

3. When you do the habit, they cheer you on or give you a high five!

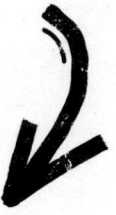

This makes you feel proud and want to keep going. And if you skip it, you might feel a little bit bad – which pushes you to try harder next time.

Some examples of how this might be helpful are:

♥ You and a friend both decide to read for ten minutes every day. You remember to talk about what you read the next day.

♥ You tell your parents that you're practising guitar every day, and they smile and clap when they hear you play.

♥ You join a team, and you don't want to skip practice because your teammates are counting on you.

This is great because connecting with other people not only makes us happy, but it also provides a way to stick to the habits that make us happy too.

PART 7: BREATHE/ REFLECT

HAPPY HABIT 13: TIME TO REFLECT

Wow! You've made it this far. Clearly, you've made a habit of reading about happy habits, and I hope you've already started to introduce some of them into your life.

We've spoken about movement and exercise, eating, resting and playing and even found time to think about how we can connect with our friends and the natural world. If you manage to do most of these things every day, I'm pretty sure you'll feel healthy and happy.

At the end of a busy day like that, can you think of the final thing you might want to do?

PAUSE. BREATHE. REFLECT.

When we reflect, we find ways to learn from all the experiences in our day. It's almost like revision for life . . . but much more pleasant! So let's think about how we reflect, why we reflect and all the ways in which it links to the happy habits we have discussed throughout the book.

So, let's start with the idea of a happy cup, which can be useful when we are reflecting on how we are feeling and thinking about what makes us happy.

FILL YOUR HAPPY CUP

Our happy cup represents our overall well-being. When we are regularly putting things in the cup that make us happy, we're happy. When we've forgotten to put things in it, and our cup is empty or only half full, we are less happy.

The thing is, many of us haven't learned how to look at our happy cup and see if it is full. It is only when we reflect that we have a chance to see what's in it, whether there is room for

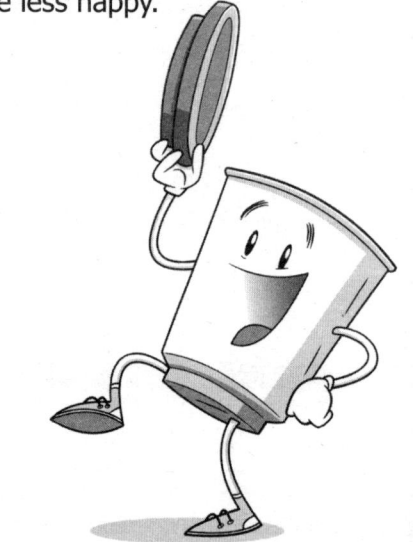

more and what might need topping up. Without reflection, our happy cup is more like a mysterious mug (with a lid).

The things that go into the cup are different for everyone. Hopefully thinking about your habits as you read this book gives you an idea of the things that make you happy. Maybe you want your cup to be full of nature, or you prefer to top it up with social time. Maybe you like a big part of your cup to be filled with movement, or you prefer it to have a big dose of creativity.

It's <u>your</u> cup, and it's your happiness, but it is only by reflecting on the things that you do that you can understand what to do tomorrow.

Whatever we enjoy, filling our happy cup involves doing lots of little things that replenish us in order to look after our mental health and to keep ourselves feeling good. It's a form of **self-care**, which means taking care of ourselves and putting our needs first. It means making ourselves the priority in our own lives when we need to.

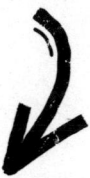

Sometimes we can count on others to do nice things to treat us and lift us up when we're struggling (or just because we deserve it). But also we need to learn to do this for ourselves as a habit that we do almost unthinkingly. Building this habit will be an intrinsic part of the well-being toolkit that we carry with us in life.

BUT ISN'T FOCUSING ON YOURSELF A BIT SELFISH?

Definitely not, but it's a common question. And it's not surprising that people get confused. There are lots of messages out there – and in this book – about the importance of thinking of others. Don't get me wrong – that is really, really important!

However, **all kindness starts from us**. And if our happy cup is empty because our needs have been neglected, then we're likely to be in a headspace where we're sad, anxious or just low on energy. And when we feel like that, it's almost impossible for us to be a source of strength and friendship to others.

So filling our happy cup is not only important for us, but it's important for those around us!

HOW DO I KNOW WHEN MY CUP NEEDS A REFILL?

We should put something into our happy cup every day, whatever's going on in our lives. Like the other habits, it should become something we do automatically once we get into the swing of it.

But it's also important to know when we really *need* it, so that we can start refilling that happy cup straight away.

This means spotting the signs that you need a break, some time alone or your favourite activity to help you recharge. We can do this by listening to our feelings as closely as we can. Feeling tired, sad or hopeless, lacking in energy, struggling to think of things to do, falling out with friends and family and feeling snappier than usual are all signs that our happy cup could probably do with a top-up.

TOP TIP

Sometimes we need to seek external help for our problems. Filling our happy cup isn't a way to replace this help, it's something extra we can do alongside it. So if things are really getting on top of you and you might need help from a trusted adult or a health professional, PLEASE REACH OUT AND ASK FOR IT.

WAYS TO TOP UP YOUR HAPPY CUP

If you look at your happy cup when your day is done and think it could use a top-up, it's always useful to know what works for you. Your happy habits are the hot chocolate in the cup – they should fill up most of it, but these top-ups are like whipped cream and sprinkles.

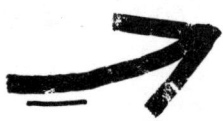

These are forms of self-care that you can introduce when you need a little burst of joy. Maybe you already know what works for you, or maybe it varies from day to day, but I'd like to give you a few suggestions that might work.

Maybe you've tried all of these, or maybe you've done none of them, so take a look, because today might be just the day your happy cup needs something new.

Here are some ideas to get you thinking:

Relax

Chill on the sofa with your favourite book or magazine! Or maybe you prefer to take a nap or just chill out listening to some music?

Dream

Write a list of your hopes and dreams, then spend some time fantasizing about what it would be like to achieve them. Don't forget to dream big!

Laugh

Watch a funny movie or plan some pranks with your funniest friend.

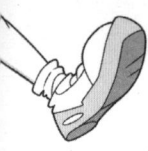

Move

Chuck your trainers on and get out of the house for a stomp or just to get some fresh air.

Bake or cook

Take the time to see if somebody could help you make yourself something delicious, then sit yourself down and enjoy it. (Whether or not you share it with others is up to you . . .)

Dance

Put on your favourite tunes and throw some shapes – in your kitchen, bedroom, wherever! It's up to you if you do this alone, with your BFF or with your siblings . . . anyone who helps you shake it all off is good to boogie with!

Create

Make something with your hands – origami, drawing, knitting, painting – come up with a story, or compose a new song. Whatever soothes you most!

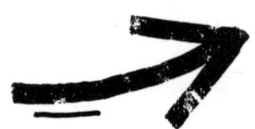

Connect

Spend time with your family. Sometimes we are so busy rushing around that we don't get a chance to just enjoy each other's company. Think about something that you and a family member both like doing, and do it *together*. This is a brilliant way of creating memories that top up your happy cup.

Read

Curl up with a good book and a hot chocolate.

Play frisbee with your dog

OK, this is quite a random one (as not everyone has a dog or enjoys playing frisbee!), but I've just included it to show that self-care really can be anything you choose as long as it recharges your batteries!

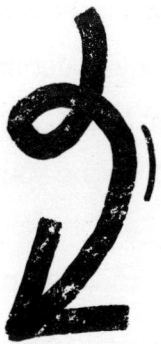

WHEN TO FILL YOUR HAPPY CUP

When to do your happy activity will depend on what it is and what else you're up to on any given day.

Often we are most capable of reflecting on our feelings later in the day, so have a think about what you feel and then decide whether the activity that will cheer you up is best for the morning or evening.

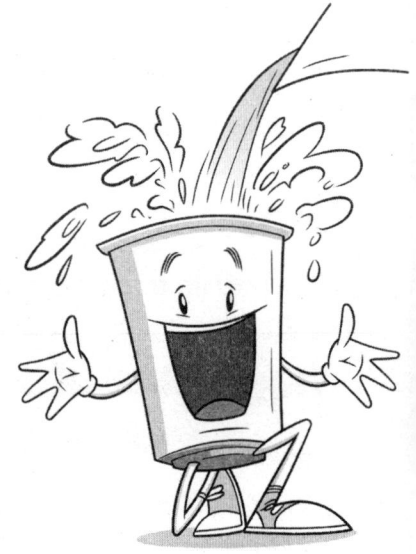

If it's late in the evening, maybe you can't go and play frisbee with your dog, but you could have a bath and get a good night's sleep before getting up early to get muddy.

Maybe you could decide that you will just have a rest and think about your happy cup over breakfast. You could even make a happy habit of thinking about your happy cup while you have your brekkie.

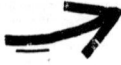

Creating this habit of just thinking about your happy activities every day at the same time means that your brain will eventually remind you to plan them as soon as you're pouring your cereal. Self-care habit formed!

JUST DO IT

I know. You weren't exactly expecting me to tell you to 'just **don't** do it', but I think we all need a reminder sometimes that all we need is a start.

So make sure you actually *do* the activity once you've planned it. Whatever else your day throws at you (extra homework, a friend who needs a chat, something unexpected popping up), try to treat it like a promise you have made to yourself and do something that's just for you (even if it's only for a bit).

There will be times when this isn't possible, and that's life. But making time for yourself despite all the hundreds of things going on around you is a wonderful, if tricky, skill to learn. It can feel hard to say 'no' to someone or cancel a plan. But if your happy cup isn't feeling full enough, it's important to choose yourself first.

KEEP A LIST

After doing a 'just for you' activity, you could make a note of it and rate it out of ten for how much it filled your happy cup. By doing this, you'll end up with a really helpful list of your favourite things, so if you're stuck for ideas one day, or too tired to think straight, you can just read over the list and choose something that's brought you joy in the past. Here's mine:

♥ Play fetch with my dog, Rolo **10/10**

♥ Listen to loud music **6/10**

♥ Run outside **10/10**

♥ Read my favourite book **7/10**

♥ Learn something new about motorbikes (mostly looking at new models and reading stats about how fast they are) **9/10**

♥ Cook my favourite meal (spag Bol) **8/10**

♥ Sit outside and people watch **6/10**

♥ Do my laundry (I love washing clothes and hanging them to dry.) **10/10**

FUTURE YOU

We'll face some challenges as we get older — that's a fact of life. If we're well-trained in looking after ourselves and keeping our happy cup full, it's the best way to make sure we're in a good headspace to tackle those challenges, whatever they may look like at any given time.

Many of the things you fill your happy cup with will change as you get older — that's normal. The habit to stay consistent with is to make sure you're doing **SOMETHING** for you every single day.

What will it be today?

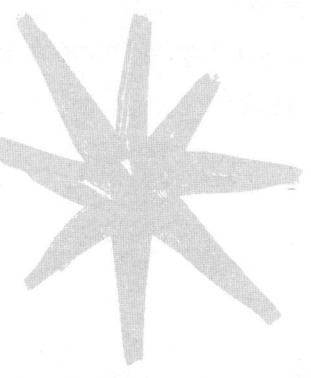

HABIT HACK: REFLECTIONS

Remember that you can reinforce your happy habits every time you reflect on your day. This is another way to give yourself a prize for the good things you have done.

So, every night before bed, stop and think about **any** of your happy habits you stuck to. Ate fruit? **Tick**. Practised my instrument? **Tick**. Homework? **Done**. This is just another way to give yourself a reward or dopamine boost.

As you go through each of them, give yourself a little tiny mini high five. This will give you a sense of achievement and you'll go to bed feeling proud, as well as encouraging you to do the same the next day.

It's a habit hack that helps your happy habits and heaps your happy cup. (That's a lot of h's. Try saying it three times, **fast**).

THE CONCLUSION

SO WE BEGIN.

I know what you're thinking – *Dr Alex, doesn't conclusion mean . . . the end?* Well, you're right. We've come to the end of this book and the end of this conversation about small changes that make a big difference.

But, really, you've only just begun.

We may be at the end of *my* book, but you are at the beginning of your journey. That journey is what we all call *life*; only I prefer to think of it as an adventure rather than a journey, and I will explain why.

A journey has a destination. There is an end-point to reach that makes the whole thing worthwhile. On a journey, we often ask, 'Are we there yet?' or 'How much further?', whereas on an adventure, well, who knows? You see, an adventure *is* the destination.

When you are on an adventure you don't know where you will end up, and you don't know quite what you will learn, but the experience is interesting.

An adventurer may not be certain of their destination, but they know each day they need to make good choices. They have to make sure their backpack is full of supplies; that they find a place to rest and prepare for the next day; and that they stay **fit**, **healthy** and **happy** as they continue going forward.

Your life is an adventure, and those good choices are your happy habits. Every time you decide to eat healthily, you are making the choice to stay fit and healthy on your adventure. A good night's sleep is not something you do because you are *meant to* but because you *want to*. When you know your life is an adventure, you want to have all the energy you need to make your discoveries. You are a **hero** and heroes don't just save the world, they eat their greens! (Superheroes eat spinach – they just don't show that bit in the movies.)

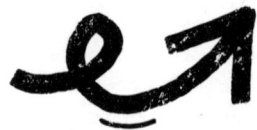

Like any good adventure, you have some idea of what you want to discover. The explorer may seek treasure, whether that's new information or new skills and abilities. **Through your adventurous life, you will find those things, and it is the habits you choose that will make you capable.**

Your treasure may be a contract at Man United. Your new information may be a great scientific discovery, or your skills and abilities could be skydiving or coding. It is good to have some idea of your goals in any adventure, but remember, it is enjoying the adventure itself that will make it worthwhile. It is your habits that will make those goals possible.

Your football practice today, tomorrow and every day until you are eighteen is what creates that contract at Man U, not the goal itself. Your habit of reading books about animals or the solar system as a child is what will make that scientific discovery happen. The way you fuel your body and mind are the steps you take up towards that bungee-jumping platform.

It won't always be easy — nothing really good ever is. The moment we learn and grow is when we try and do something that feels too hard, that then begins to seem possible and *finally* becomes easy. This is often the way with happy habits.

There is a bit of a struggle at the start, like a child learning the shapes of letters (with their tongue sticking out, concentrating *soooo* hard). Then there is a time when you realize you don't even need to think about the shape, but you need to do a bit of work to remember how to spell the words. Then, the spelling (which was hard) becomes easy, and now the challenge is creating good paragraphs, then essays, then books.

The hard bit is the sign that you are growing to another level. **The challenging time *is* the progress.** Any time you are struggling with a habit, just remember that you are doing it *just right* – you are overcoming the final boss before the next level.

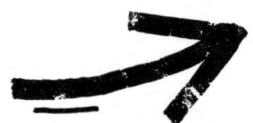

This becomes easier to appreciate as we move along. Once we have got past a hard part and felt our progress a few times, we begin to realize that it is a necessary part of learning. So remember that the *hardest hard part* will probably be at the very beginning, before you have learned how helpful the challenge is.

So, stick with your habits at the very beginning. Make a habit of sticking it out, if only to learn that you can. Remind yourself that the hard part at the beginning is *exactly* what will make the next part easier. The first days of a habit are like learning letters, but in the future, you'll be writing books.

Remember that **these habits are all for you.** Your parents might praise you for making good choices; your friends might notice that you are able to run faster or remember more dance moves; and you might start winning prizes that you never expected to get. Good habits really do create results like that, but those results are not the reason.

Your habits may make other people feel good about you, but all that matters is that they make you feel good *within yourself.* If you can make a habit of giving yourself a high five when you do well, speaking kindly to yourself when you are sad, or giving yourself a pep talk when you need some encouragement, you will have learned a skill for a lifetime. You will have made a habit of happy habits, which is a habit for life.

There are many adults who have never learned this. They spend their whole lives doing things so other people say well done or give them money. Then, one day, they realize that the one person who never thought 'well done' was themselves. **So focus on making *yourself* proud of you.** Celebrate your habits and forgive your own mistakes and you will have learned the secret of a fun and adventurous life.

I don't know which habits from this book will appeal to you. Maybe you will learn some from friends or discover some of your own. (If you do, get your mum or dad to send me a comment on Instagram! I want to learn from *you*).

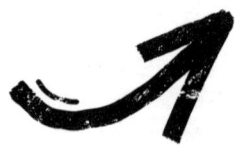

We never know where we will go or what we will learn in this life, and that's what makes it an adventure. So don't worry about preparing for the future – just take care of yourself today, and it will all work out fine.

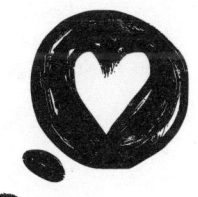

IF YOUR HABITS ARE HAPPY, YOU WILL BE TOO - WHEREVER YOUR ADVENTURE TAKES YOU!

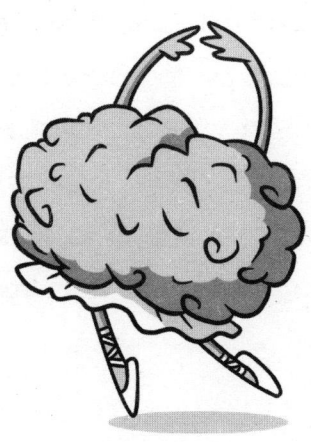

LETTER FROM DR. ALEX

Dear reader,

There you have it: the happy habits that helped me build the life I live.

All I have given you are the tools, so it's your choice what you want to build. Your life and the habits that make it are yours to choose and yours to shape into the form that reflects you. Maybe it will become a tower of creativity, a great sprawling mass of scientific discovery or a field of footballing dreams.

I hope my guide has helped you appreciate these building blocks and motivated you to create something great. You deserve it.

Most of all, you deserve to be happy, to do things that make you feel good and achieve things that make you feel proud.

Once you start, you'll find they have their own power to keep you going. They start as happy habits that we practise and learn, but soon just become part of our everyday happy life.

So learn, build and grow. Then let me know about what you create. The dreams that come true. The habits which make you happy.

I believe in you.

Dr Alex

REFERENCES

Children's physical activity
Coe, D.P. et al. (2006) 'Effect of physical education and activity levels on academic achievement in children', *Medicine & Science in Sports & Exercise*, 38(8), pp. 1515–1519. doi:10.1249/01.mss.0000227537.13175.1b.

de Greeff, J.W. et al. (2014) 'Physical fitness and academic performance in primary school children with and without a social disadvantage', *Health Education Research*, 29(5), pp. 853–860. doi:10.1093/her/cyu043.

Escalante, Y. et al. (2011) 'Relationship between daily physical activity, recess physical activity, age and sex in scholar of primary school, Spain', *Revista Española de Salud Pública*, 85(5), pp. 481–489. doi:10.1590/S1135-57272011000500007.

Hallal, P.C. et al. (2012) 'Global physical activity levels: surveillance progress, pitfalls, and prospects', *The Lancet*, 380(9838), pp. 247–257. doi:10.1016/S0140-6736(12)60646-1.

Janssen, I. and LeBlanc, A.G. (2010) 'Systematic review of the health benefits of physical activity and fitness in school-aged children and youth', *International Journal of Behavioral Nutrition and Physical Activity*, 7(40). doi:10.1186/1479-5868-7-40.

Strong, W.B. et al. (2005) 'Evidence based physical activity for school-age youth', *The Journal of Pediatrics*, 146(6), pp. 732–737. doi:10.1016/j.jpeds.2005.01.055.

Cognitive Benefits of Exercise on Children
Liu, S. et al. (2020) 'Effects of Acute and Chronic Exercises on Executive Function in Children and Adolescents: A Systemic Review and Meta-Analysis', *Frontiers in Psychology*, 11, 554915. doi: 10.3389/fpsyg.2020.554915.

Purgato M. et al. (2024), 'Umbrella Systematic Review and Meta-Analysis: Physical Activity as an Effective Therapeutic Strategy for Improving Psychosocial Outcomes in Children and Adolescents.' *Journal of the American Academy of Child and Adolescent Psychiatry*, 2024 Feb. doi: 10.1016/j.jaac.2023.04.017.

Singh, A.S. et al. (2019), 'Effects of physical activity interventions on cognitive and academic performance in children and adolescents: a novel combination of a systematic review and recommendations from an expert panel', *British Journal of Sports Medicine*, 53(10), pp. 640–647. doi: 10.1136/bjsports-2017-098136.

Vazou S. et al. (2019) 'More than one road leads to Rome: A narrative review and meta-analysis of physical activity intervention effects on cognition in youth', *Int J Sport Exerc Psychol*. 2019;17(2):153-178. doi: 10.1080/1612197X.2016.1223423.

The Value of Maintaining Streaks
Aulagnon, R. et al. (2024) 'Streaking to success: The effects of highlighting streaks on student effort and learning', *IBD Working Paper Series*. doi: 10.18235/0012912.

Curran, M. et al. (2024) 'Look, over there! A streaker! – Qualitative study examining streaking as a behaviour change technique for habit formation in recreational runners', *Health Psychology and Behavioral Medicine*, 12(1). doi: 10.1080/21642850.2024.2416505.

Silverman, J., Barasch, A.P. and Small, D.A. (2023) 'Hot streak! Inferences and predictions about goal adherence', *Organizational Behavior and Human Decision Processes*, 179, 104281. doi: 10.1016/j.obhdp.2023.104281. Available at: https://www.sciencedirect.com/science/article/pii/S0749597823000572. (Accessed: 30 May 2025).

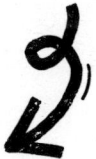

Intuitive Eating

Babbott K.M. et al. (2023) 'Outcomes of intuitive eating interventions: a systematic review and meta-analysis', *Eating Disorders*, 31(1), pp. 33–63. doi: 10.1080/10640266.2022.2030124.

Clean Spaces and Wellbeing

Hanley, A.W. et al. (2015) 'Washing dishes to wash the dishes: Brief instruction in an informal mindfulness practice', *Mindfulness*, 6(5), pp. 1095–1103. doi:10.1007/s12671-014-0360-9.

McMains, S. and Kastner, S. (2011) 'Interactions of top-down and bottom-up mechanisms in human visual cortex', *The Journal of Neuroscience*, 31(2), pp. 587–597. doi:10.1523/JNEUROSCI.3766-10.2011.

Roster, C.A., Ferrari, J.R. and Jurkat, M.P. (2016) 'The dark side of home: Assessing possession "clutter" on subjective well-being', *Journal of Environmental Psychology*, 46, pp. 32–41. doi:10.1016/j.jenvp.2016.03.003.

Saxbe, D.E. and Repetti, R.L. (2010) 'No place like home: Home tours correlate with daily patterns of mood and cortisol', *Personality and Social Psychology Bulletin*, 36(1), pp. 71–81. doi:10.1177/0146167209352864.

Non-linear Progress through Habit Formation

Carroll, C.D., Overland, J. and Weil, D.N. (2000) 'Saving and growth with habit formation', *American Economic Review*, 90(3), pp. 341–355. doi: 10.1257/aer.90.3.341.

Lally, P. et al. (2010) 'How are habits formed: Modelling habit formation in the real world', *European Journal of Social Psychology*, 40(6), pp. 998–1009. doi: 10.1002/ejsp.674.

Yamada, K. and Toda, K. (2023) 'Habit formation viewed as structural change in the behavioral network', *Communications Biology*, 6(303). doi: 10.1038/s42003-023-04500-2.

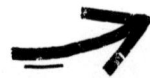

Sun Exposure and Children
Salvado, M. et al. (2021) 'Sun Exposure in Pediatric Age: Perspective of Caregivers', *Children*, 8(11), p. 1019. doi: 10.3390/children8111019.

Reading and Stress
Levine SL. et al. (2022) 'For the love of reading: Recreational reading reduces psychological distress in college students and autonomous motivation is the key'. *J Am Coll Health*. 2022 Jan;70(1):158-164. doi: 10.1080/07448481.2020.1728280. Epub 2020 Mar 9. PMID: 32150516.

Mak HW. et al. (2020) 'Reading for pleasure in childhood and adolescent healthy behaviours: Longitudinal associations using the Millennium Cohort Study'. *Preventative Medicine*. 2020 Jan;130:105889. doi: 10.1016/j.ypmed.2019.105889. Epub 2019 Nov 23. PMID: 31765711; PMCID: PMC6983940.

Children and Smartphones
Haidt, J. (2024) *The Anxious Generation: How the Great Rewiring of Childhood Is Causing an Epidemic of Mental Illness*. New York: Penguin Press.

Willpower and Smartphones
de Werd D. et al.(2018) 'Why is the smartphone such a distraction – even when not actively used?', Tilburg University. Available at: arno.uvt.nl/show.cgi?fid=152372. (Accessed: 30/5/2025).

Figueroa, C. et al. (2018) 'FamilyTime: How to help smartphone users reduce problematic smartphone behaviour', London School of Economics and Political Science. Available at: https://www.lse.ac.uk/PBS/assets/documents/FamilyTime-How-to-help-smartphone-users-reduce-problematic-smartphone-behaviour.pdf. (Accessed: 30/5/2025).

Zhu, Y., Chen, J., and Zhang, E. (2023) 'Understanding and addressing smartphone addiction: A multidisciplinary perspective', *Journal of Addiction Medicine and Therapeutic Science*, 9(1), pp. 1–4. doi: 10.17352/2455-3484.000055. Available at: https://www.neuroscigroup.us/articles/JAMTS-9-155.pdf.

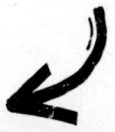

Hours of Daily Screen Time UK
Bennett, A. (2024) 'The State of Screen Time in the United Kingdom', Opal. www.opal.so/blog/the-state-of-screen-time-in-the-uk. (Accessed: 30/5/2025).

Nature, Cognition and Wellbeing
Chang, C. et al (2024) Pritchard, A., Richardson, M., Sheffield, D. and McEwan, K. (2024) 'A lower connection to nature is linked to lower mental health benefits from nature contact', *Scientific Reports*, 14, 6705. doi: 10.1038/s41598-024-56968-5. Available at: www.nature.com/articles/s41598-024-56968-5. (Accessed: 19 May 2025).

McDonnell, A.S. et al. (2024), Strayer, D.L. 'The influence of a walk in nature on human resting brain activity: a randomized controlled trial', *Scientific Reports*, 14, 27253. doi: 10.1038/s41598-024-78508-x. Available at: www.nature.com/articles/s41598-024-78508-x. (Accessed: 19 May 2025).

Rhee, J.H. et al. (2023) 'Effects of nature on restorative and cognitive benefits in indoor environment', *Scientific Reports*, 13, 13199. doi: 10.1038/s41598-023-40408-x. Available at: www.nature.com/articles/s41598-023-40408-x. (Accessed: 19 May 2025).

Sudimac, S. et al. (2022), 'How nature nurtures: Amygdala activity decreases as the result of a one-hour walk in nature', *Mol Psychiatry* 27, 4446–4452 https://doi.org/10.1038/s41380-022-01720-6 (Accessed: 19 May 2025).

Sudimac, S. and Kühn, S. (2024) 'Can a nature walk change your brain? Investigating hippocampal brain plasticity after one hour in a forest', *Environmental Research*, 262(1). doi: 10.1016/j.envres.2024.119813. Available at: www.sciencedirect.com/science/article/pii/S0013935124017183 (Accessed: 19 May 2025).

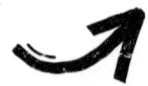

Friendship and Wellbeing

Bagwell, C.L. & Schmidt, M.E. (2011) *Friendships in Childhood and Adolescence*. Guilford Press.

Holt-Lunstad, J., Smith, T.B. and Layton, J.B. (2010) 'Social relationships and mortality risk: A meta-analytic review', *PLoS Medicine*, 7(7), e1000316. doi:10.1371/journal.pmed.1000316.

Scheuplein, M. and van Harmelen, A. L. (2022) 'The importance of friendships in reducing brain responses to stress in adolescents exposed to childhood adversity: a preregistered systematic review.', *Current Opinion in Psychology*, 45, 101310. doi: 10.1016/j.copsyc.2022.101310.

Steptoe, A. et al. (2013) 'Social isolation, loneliness, and all-cause mortality in older men and women', *Proceedings of the National Academy of Sciences*, 110(15), pp. 5797–5801. doi:10.1073/pnas.1219686110.

Studies on Accountability in Habit Formation

Chhabria K. et al. (2020) 'The assessment of supportive accountability in adults seeking obesity treatment: Psychometric validation study', *Journal of Medical Internet Research*, 22(7), e17967. doi: 10.2196/17967. Available at: www.ncbi.nlm.nih.gov/pmc/articles/PMC7420735/. (Accessed: 30/05/2025).

Feil, K. et al. (2021) 'A systematic review examining the relationship between habit strength and physical activity behavior in longitudinal studies', *Frontiers in Psychology*, 12, 626750. doi: 10.3389/fpsyg.2021.626750. Available at: www.frontiersin.org/articles/10.3389/fpsyg.2021.626750/full. (Accessed: 30/5/2025).

Salisbury, K.R., Ranpariya, V.K. and Feldman, S.R. (2022) 'Accountability in reminder-based adherence interventions: A review', *Patient Education and Counseling*, 105(8), pp. 2645–2652. doi: 10.1016/j.pec.2021.12.009. Available at: www.sciencedirect.com/science/article/abs/pii/S0738399121007862. (Accessed: 30/5/2025).

ACKNOWLEDGEMENTS

I would say that I have experienced a wide range of emotions in my life – from moments of absolute joy through to sadness and despair. What I've learned is that no high is possible, and no low surmountable, without the love and affection of the people I call family. Some of those people I was born with, and others have joined along the way. To all of you, I would like to say thank you and I love you dearly.

This book is everything I dreamed of and more. To my wonderful team (and friends) Harry Grenville, Carly Cook, Abby Wagge, Immy Rooney and Susanna Kidd – I am so grateful for you all.

To Fenella Bates, Emma Young, Pippa Shaw, Kat McKenna, Sophia Pringle and the rest of the team at Penguin Random House, thank you for helping me create a book that every child needs to read.

A big thank you to Oscar Millar for going over and above, I am lucky to work with you.

To those who support and love me unconditionally, you know who you are, and I am forever grateful. I love you always.